www.harcourt-international.com

Bringing you products from all Harcourt Health Sciences companies including Baillière Tindall, Churchill Livingstone, Mosby and W.B. Saunders

- ● **Browse** for latest information on new books, journals and electronic products

- ● **Search** for information on over 20 000 published titles with full product information including tables of contents and sample chapters

- ● **Keep up to date** with our extensive publishing programme in your field by registering with eAlert or requesting postal updates

- ● **Secure online ordering** with prompt delivery, as well as full contact details to order by phone, fax or post

- ● **News** of special features and promotions

If you are based in the following countries, please visit the country-specific site to receive full details of product availability and local ordering information

USA: www.harcourthealth.com

Canada: www.harcourtcanada.com

Australia: www.harcourt.com.au

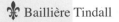

Baillière Tindall   CHURCHILL LIVINGSTONE   Mosby   W.B. SAUNDERS

The Nurse's Handbook of Complementary Therapies

Edited by

Denise Rankin-Box BA(Hons) RGN DipTD CertED MISMA
Freelance Consultant, Macclesfield, UK;
Editor, *Complementary Therapies in Nursing and Midwifery*

SECOND EDITION

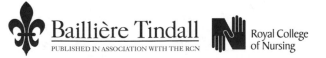

Baillière Tindall
PUBLISHED IN ASSOCIATION WITH THE RCN

Royal College
of Nursing

EDINBURGH LONDON NEW YORK PHILADELPHIA ST LOUIS SYDNEY TORONTO 2001

BAILLIÈRE TINDALL
An imprint of Harcourt Publishers Limited

© Harcourt Publishers Limited 2001

✿ is a registered trademark of Harcourt Publishers Limited

The right of Denise Rankin-Box to be identified as editor of this work
has been asserted by her in accordance with the Copyright, Designs
and Patents Act 1988

First published 2001
  Reprinted 2001

ISBN 0 7020 2651 4

British Library Cataloguing in Publication Data
A catalogue record for this book is available from the British Library

Library of Congress Cataloging in Publication Data
A catalog record for this book is available from the Library of
Congress

Note
Medical knowledge is constantly changing. As new information
becomes available, changes in treatment, procedures, equipment and
the use of drugs become necessary. The editors, contributors and the
publishers have taken care to ensure that the information given in this
text is accurate and up to date. However, readers are strongly advised
to confirm that the information, especially with regard to drug usage,
complies with the latest legislation and standards of practice.

The
publisher's
policy is to use
paper manufactured
from sustainable forests

Printed in China by RDC Group Limited

Contents

Contributors

Kenneth Atherton FSBiolMed RGN BRCP (Classical Hom)
LFHom DiplomaEAV VEGACert(Germany)
Medical Homeopath; NHS/University Lecturer, Merseyside, UK

Angela Avis MA RGN DNCert PGDipEd PGDip(Advanced Health Care Practice)
Senior Lecturer, School of Health Care, Oxford Brookes University, Oxford, UK; Chair, Royal College of Nursing Complementary Therapies Forum, UK

Daniel J Benor MD
Psychiatrist and Spiritual Healer,
Medford, New Jersey, USA

Ruth Benor RGN RM RHV RNT DCertEd DipAT UKCPRegCounsCert
Senior Lecturer in Palliative Care,
Devon, UK

Francis C Biley PhD MSc BNurs RN PGCE FETCert
Senior Lecturer, University of Wales College of Medicine,
Cardiff, UK

David Bray DC
Private Practitioner, Leeds, UK

Helen Busby MSc
Doctoral researcher, University of Nottingham, Nottingham, UK

Clare Byrne MSc BA(Hons) RGN
Advanced Nurse Practitioner,
Royal Liverpool University Hospital Trust, Liverpool, UK

Anne Cawthorn BSc(Hons) DipN RGN OND CertCouns CertEd MISPA
Lecturer/Practitioner, Christie Hospital
and Manchester University, Manchester, UK

Dorothy Crowther BSc RGN RCNT RNT FRCN
Chief Executive,
Wirral Holistic Therapeutic Cancer Centre,
Birkenhead, UK

Brian Daniels MIPR
Head of Communications, General Osteopathic Council, London, UK

Stephanie Downey MSc BA(Hons) RGN BAc MBAcC
Co-Director, Brighton Acupuncture Centre, Brighton, UK

Dawn Freshwater PhD BA(Hons) RNT RGN
Senior Research Fellow, Mary Seacole Research Centre, De Montfort University, Leicester

Pamela Griffiths BA RGN ONC RCNT RNT CertEd
Home, Manager, Peniel Green, Cardiff, UK

Carol Horrigan MSc SRN DipN RCNT PGCEA RNT
Independent Nurse Consultant and Educator in Complementary Therapies,
Myall Mundy, Queensland, Australia

Brian Isbell PhD MRN DO MIBiol CBiol BSc
Osteopath and Naturopath; Director of Undergraduate Studies, School of Integrated Health, University of Westminster, London, UK

Peter A Mackereth MA RGN RNT
Nurse Teacher/Research Associate, School of Nursing, Midwifery and Health Visiting, University of Manchester, Manchester, UK

Maxine McVey MN RN
Service Manager, Surgical Department, West Hertfordshire Hospitals NHS Trust, Hemel Hempstead, UK

Jane Mallett PhD MSc BSc RN
Nursing and Rehabilitation Research and Development Manager, The Royal Marsden Hospital, London, UK

Fiona Mantle BSc(Hons) RN RHV CertEd RNT
Senior Lecturer, Oxford Brookes University, Oxford, UK

Mike Money PhD MA BA(Hons) DipEd AFBPsS CPsychol
Principal Lecturer/Centre Academic Manager, Centre for Health, Healing and Human Development, School of Health and Human Sciences, Liverpool John Moores University, Liverpool

Denise Rankin-Box BA(Hons) RGN DipTD CertEd
Freelance Consultant, Macclesfield, UK;
Editor, *Complementary Therapies in Nursing and Midwifery*

Lynne Ryman RGN ONC NFSH
formerly Relaxation Therapist, The Royal Marsden Hospital,
London, UK

Jean Sayre-Adams MA RN
Director, The Sacred Space Foundation, Cumbria

Caroline Stevensen BSW RGN DipAc MRSS MIFA LFHom(Nurse)
Senior Lecturer (Clinical Aromatherapy), Oxford Brookes
University, Oxford, UK;
Holistic Health Consultant and Practitioner, London, UK

Julie Stone
Senior Lecturer in Health Care Ethics and Law,
School of Health, University of Greenwich, London

Steven G Wright MSc RN DipN RCNT RNT DANS RPTT FRCN MBE
Chairman, The Scared Space Foundation, Cumbria;
Associate Professor, Faculty of Health, St Martin's College,
Lancaster

Foreword to the first edition

This handbook of complementary therapy for nurses is both timely and interesting. It is a valuable resource for nurses who are actively involved in using complementary therapy, and those who are interested in expanding their practice to offer greater choice to patients and clients.

In recent years, there has been growing pressure on nurses to prove their value in terms of their cost effectiveness and their contribution to patient well being. Nurses have accepted this challenge, proving that qualified nursing care not only helps people to get better quicker, but in the long term, it actually costs less.

One of the most important aspects of nursing's contribution is the added value it brings to the health care team. Nurses bring a new dimension to care, increasing the variety as well as the volume and the quality of care available.

Based on a growing confidence of this value, nurses everywhere are pushing at the boundaries of care to find innovative ways of solving long standing problems. The increased use and greater understanding of complementary therapies provides a good example of this.

Nurses understand the importance of basing their practice on experience and research. Nursing research enables them to ensure that innovative practice really does enhance the quality of care that patients receive. At the same time, for nursing to continue to develop as a flourishing, autonomous, practice-based discipline, it must be replenished and strengthened by the new knowledge and new insights derived from research.

Nurses also understand that changing the way things are done can cause its own difficulties. Introducing complementary therapies into practice requires a cautious and sensitive approach with colleagues and patients alike.

Thus, the handbook's exploration of research issues and how to choose and manage a therapy is invaluable.

The handbook includes a comprehensive introduction to many of the therapies used by nurses today and the way in which they are being applied in a range of settings.

As such, the handbook is an excellent working guide, and a constructive tool in the wider and continuing debate on the value of nursing.

London 1995   Christine Hancock

Preface

It is with great delight that I write the preface to this new expanded edition of the Nurse's Handbook. When the book was first published in 1995, it was apparent that interest in complementary therapies, both in the lay and health care arenas, was expanding at a tremendous rate. The intervening years have borne witness to greater consolidation and awareness of the potential for the use of complementary medicine (CM) within current health care practice. Under the patronage of HRH Prince of Wales, the Foundation for Integrated Medicine (FIM), established in 1993, is now perceived as pivotal in the promotion of research, development, education, regulation and delivery mechanisms in the UK today. There are now more than 20 universities in the UK offering a range of undergraduate and postgraduate modules and courses in aspects of this field.

Since the first edition was published, I have become increasingly aware of a subtle yet significant shift in the way people view complementary therapies. There is a growing awareness that the efficacy of a therapy may not be solely reliant upon specific techniques or procedures but may also be influenced by *how* therapeutic care is given and the *context* in which this occurs. This has recently been referred to as the 'therapeutic relationship' or 'encounter'.

Although the processes by which therapies such as homeopathy or acupuncture work are still uncertain, it may be that we have yet to recognize and understand finer, more subtle aspects of healing. Discovering hitherto untapped resources is, however, part of the evolution of scientific discovery on our planet. Electricity, for example, was initially hailed as a passing fad that would never catch on and, like many complementary therapies, only the *effects* of electricity can be seen.

Despite the sheer range of therapies on offer today, there often appear to be similarities between therapies, leading us to question whether therapies are merely techniques that enable us to 'tap' into some fundamental form of healing. Diverse as therapies appear to be, perhaps they are like drops of water. Depending upon the environment, transformations occur creating variations in form and appearance; thus, water can also present as vapour, fog, cloud, ice, hail, snow, icebergs or great continents of ice. Individual snow flakes appear to carry with them an ability to create incredible symmetrical shapes. Varying perceptions of each form alter our use of, and response to, what is fundamentally one element – water. Thus the multitude of therapies in practice may also represent alternate perceptions of a fundamental healing process.

This book has been carefully compiled and expanded with these shifts in our perceptions of health care in mind.

Integrating complementary therapies within the workplace necessitates managing change – merging the best of the old world order towards an improved new health era. Thus, Section 1 of the book includes chapters on key practical issues, including policy development, research, clinical supervision, managing change and ethicolegal issues.

A completely new second section has been developed to stimulate discussion and an awareness of the influence of other factors that contribute to the healing process. New chapters highlight a range of concepts in relation to current health care that have not been fully explored before in one text. These include sacred space, hospitals as healing environments, shamanism and how we learn from other cultures.

The final therapy section has been expanded and updated to provide a concise introduction to therapies currently in use today. Potential indications, contraindications for use and research evidence have also been addressed. Contact names and addresses are provided should you wish to explore a particular therapy further.

As with the first edition, my aim is that this book should be a working text – write in it, add telephone numbers, make notes in the margin and let it get curly at the edges. It is to be used and flicked through – a working text and guide to facilitate your future studies and exploration of innovative forms of health care. Alternatively simply read and enjoy! If there are additional issues you would like to have included in future editions, let me know.

To my knowledge, this is the *only* book in the field of complementary medicine that draws together practice, philosophy, spirituality, research, therapeutic approaches, law and ethics, policy development, and healing environments under one cover. Even now the list of topics is not exhaustive but that is the nature of evolution – social values shift. The mission to enhance health and well-being will take us on a long journey – a journey of discovery. It may be that in the not so distant future we might glean greater insight into some of the broader more complex processes of our universe, health and healing.

As Carl Sagan (1980) commented:

> Lost somewhere between immensity and eternity is our tiny planetary home. In a cosmic perspective, most human concerns seems insignificant, even petty. And yet our species is young and curious and brave and shows much promise. In the last few millennia we have made the most astonishing and unexpected discoveries about the cosmos ... They remind us that humans have evolved to wonder, that understanding is a joy, that knowledge is a prerequisite to survival. I believe that our future depends on how well we know this Cosmos in which we float like a mote of dust in the morning sky.

I hope this book takes you a little further along the road of discovery.

Prestbury 2001   Denise Rankin-Box

Reference
Sagan C 1980 Cosmos. Book Club Associates, USA, p 4

Acknowledgements

My grateful thanks to all the contributors for their time and commitment in this endeavor – it was greatly appreciated. I am also grateful to Inta Ozols of Harcourt, for offering me the opportunity to undertake an expanded edition of the Handbook so that it could evolve and reflect current developments in this field.

Special thanks to my husband Ian for his love, support and for providing the time to undertake this project. To our daughters, Carla and Felicity, who continue to share with me their unique way of perceiving the world.

Heartfelt thanks also go to some special friends for simply being there: Sue and John, Vicky and Chris, and Sue and Pete—*ginger nuts for the soul*, supper parties and a lot of giggles that put the world into a new perspective!

Denise Rankin-Box, 2001

1 Introduction

Denise Rankin-Box

'It is one of the commonest of mistakes to consider that the limit of our power of perception is also the limit of all there is to perceive'
C W Leadbeater

Complementary therapies in health care are not new. The use of herbs, oils, laying on of hands or the treatment of forms of energy within the human body appear to have existed in some form or another for thousands of years. Complementary therapies do not represent a rediscovery of therapeutic forms of healing – peoples in tribes and multifarious cultures around the world have continued to use natural forms of health care and ritualized approaches to healing over the centuries. Indeed there has never been a time when many of the therapies described in this handbook have not been in existence somewhere in human history. However, the social recognition afforded to certain therapies and reliance placed upon their efficacy appears to have shifted over time.

Social trends and cultural change similarly influence a person's health care beliefs. As a result, some health care practices such as herbalism or healing have been the object of ridicule and persecution during certain periods of social history. Perhaps current health care trends demanding choice in health care treatment are simply social trends and a response to consumer desire in the search for the 'panacea for all ills'.

Interestingly the shift towards individualized forms of health care is not only occurring in one small area of Western society but, according to the British Medical Association (BMA), a number of indicators suggests that there has been an increase in the use of non-conventional therapies not only in the UK but also in the US and in Europe (BMA 1993, Eisenberg et al 1993, Stone 1999).

CAM IN EUROPE AND THE US

Trevelyan (1998) notes that in Europe, the status of complementary therapies varies. In the Netherlands, Germany or Denmark for example, non-conventional medicine is practised within 'certain limits'.

However in Southern countries, including France, Belgium and Luxembourg, only the medical profession is entitled to practise health care and treat illnesses (Trevelyan 1998).

In 1994 the European Parliament's Committee on the Environment Public Health and Consumer Protection acknowledged a report by MEP Paul Lannoye which sought to establish a principle of plurality on medicine through the regulation and recognition of complementary medicine. Trevelyan (1998) noted that this included the regulation and training of complementary practitioners by harmonizing the training and legal status in each member state. In 1997 an amended report was accepted by the European Commission; however, more research has been requested into a number of issues including safety and efficacy.

Even allowing for greater communication across nations using current technology it is not easy to explain the current explosion of interest in the use of complementary medicine in health care. In part, there may be disillusionment with the perceived limitations of reductionist forms of medicine and the apparent failure to treat and/or cure chronic illness and catastrophic disease such as cancer or AIDS.

To some extent, disquiet focusing upon the failures of modern medicine is a little misplaced. Whilst a number of medical 'breakthroughs' might appear to be a little like taking a sledgehammer to crack a nut, many other developments have undoubtedly wrought modern-day miracles in the management of illness. Ironically, it could be that current systems of medical practice have been hoisted by their own petard – the very successes enhancing health and extending longevity have given birth to a new generation of illnesses and dilemmas previously limited by shorter lifespans.

Stone (1999a) has commented that the disillusionment which is often voiced in relation to orthodox medicine is directed primarily towards the reductionist, biomedical model which views patients more in terms of symptoms than as a whole person. In other words, she suggests, it is the medical culture which is found wanting, not necessarily the personnel who attempt to deliver health care (Stone 1999a).

Additionally, the successful use of preventive medicine and enhanced quality of health in the West has resulted in an increasingly critical reflection of the way in which health and illness is perceived and care meted out when treating disorders. There is growing recognition of the interplay between mind and body upon the state of an individual's health and wellbeing. This has resulted in the recognition of the process of care as well as the outcome and the role of the therapeutic relationship in facilitating the healing process.

Within nursing practice the nature of care provided for a client is dependent upon some form of therapeutic relationship. This was described by Hockey 'as the practice of those nursing activities which have a healing effect or those which result in a movement towards health or wellness' (Hockey 1991). The use of complementary therapies within nursing practice not only builds upon this approach to care but seeks to utilize nursing practice in a specific way – to proactively negotiate and facilitate the healing process using specific therapeutic procedures. Such an approach is challenging and innovative since it obviates generalistic approaches to current models of nursing laying claim to highly individualized systems of health care based upon a case-load approach. The increasing use of complementary therapies in nursing and midwifery raises issues associated with competence and efficacy. This in turn directs attention towards education and training in complementary and alternative medicine (CAM) and ethical considerations promoting client safety and protecting nurses engaged in the practice of CAM.

In the UK, approximately 4–5 million people a year consult complementary practitioners and in the USA an estimated $15 *billion* per annum is spent on complementary therapies with approximately one in four of the population using some aspect of complementary therapy (Eisenberg et al 1993, Stone 1999a). Indeed, Fulder and Monro (1985) established that 13 million visits to 7500 practitioners of complementary medicine took place annually in the UK as early as 1980–1981 (Harris 1995).

Nurses, midwives and health visitors collectively represent the largest group of National Health Service (NHS) employees (DHS 1993). However, to date, the actual numbers of nurses practising complementary therapies within the NHS or in private practice has not been quantified.

EDUCATION AND TRAINING IN THE UK

In the UK, non-medically qualified practitioners of CAM are free to practise under common law, irrespective of their levels of training or clinical competence. Practitioners are subject only to the relevant provisions of statutes such as the Medical, Dental, Professions Supplementary to Medicine and Medicines Acts (FIM 1997).

Despite much talk about the integration of complementary and orthodox medicine in the UK, developments towards standardizing education, training and practice take time. As Stone (1999a) comments, 'the pace of integration at any meaningful level is slow, and still depends to a large extent on the enthusiasm of committed individuals' (Stone 1999a, p. 2).

In 1997 the Foundation for Integrated Medicine (FIM) produced a key report in the field of CAM entitled, 'Integrated healthcare: a way forward for the next five years'. The report outlined the results of four working parties addressing central issues associated with the integration of CAM within health care – research and development, education and training, regulation and delivery mechanisms.

The aim of the Education and Training working party was to consider how best to encourage and support the development of a common core curriculum providing a common foundation for all health care training, both orthodox and complementary; to support specialist CAM training and continuing professional training for all health care practitioners; finally to encourage and promote better information on CAM for both patients and health care practitioners (FIM 1997).

UKKC AND CAM EDUCATION

As far back as 1992, the United Kingdom Central Council (UKCC) revised their advisory paper, 'Administration of medicines' and recognized for the first time the growing use of complementary therapies within nursing practice (Rankin-Box 1995). Paragraphs 38 and 39 referred explicitly to the administration of herbal, homeopathic and CAM.

With reference to complementary therapies the UKCC is keen to point out that, whilst it regulates the nursing, midwifery and health-visiting professions, it does not have a responsibility for the standards of other bodies which offer education and training in professional or complementary therapies (Knape 1998). However, the standards required by the UKCC of all registrants apply during the use of CAM as at all other times. These requirements are set out in the Code of Professional Conduct (UKCC 1992).

ABOUT THIS BOOK

Although there has been a great expansion of interest, research and publishing in the field of complementary medicine there has been little attempt to highlight a number of practical issues associated with the formal development and integration of complementary therapies within the workplace. Additionally, whilst many books testify to the benefits of specific therapies, in general, texts do not focus upon the use and implications certain therapies may have with immunocompromised clients and so indications and contraindications of use are not clearly presented. The aim of this book was to try to go some way to resolving these dilemmas for nurses wishing to include certain therapies in nursing practice. I was also keen to expand this edition to include a more in-depth reflection of the concept of the healing spirit. Approaches to healing include a number of perspectives on this topic with the aim of encouraging readers to reflect upon the nature and context of healing – in essence an approach not confined to complementary therapies but a perspective and way of perceiving life in general.

The topics and therapies selected for inclusion are those that nurses had expressed an interest in, to me, and come not only from the UK but also the US, Canada, Israel and Australia. Knowing about therapies is not enough; for this approach to become successfully integrated into mainstream nursing practice, protocol development, managing change, research and spiritual awareness are essential.

The aim was to develop a user-friendly handbook that nurses could carry around with them designed in such a way as to provide easy access to any part of the handbook. I hope we have gone some way to meeting this need.

As nursing practice continues to evolve, reflect and dynamically shape health care trends in society, so more therapies and associated administrative issues will come to the fore and a second handbook will become necessary. Clearly developments in this field of care should not be perceived as exclusive to nursing care. Close collaboration across the professional health care spectrum can only serve to promote and integrate complementary medicine within orthodox practice. Additionally, initiating professional debate concerning treatment efficacy, the substantive base of certain therapies and the issues of educational competence reinforces the proactive stance that the nursing profession is willing to adopt in order to provide a therapeutic partnership in care.

As we begin to question current perceptions of health and illness we should also begin to ask questions about the general way in which we perceive these. Indeed, as Reilly and Taylor suggest, 'proof is more often demanded than defined' (Reilly & Taylor 1993).

REFERENCES

BMA 1993 Complementary medicine: new approaches to good practice. British Medical Association / Oxford University Press, Oxford

Eisenberg D et al 1993 Unconventional medicine in the United States. Prevalence, costs and patterns of use. New England Journal of Medicine 328: 246–252

FIM 1997 Integrated healthcare: a way forward for the next five years? A Discussion Document. FIM, London

Fulder S Monro R E 1985 Complementary medicine in the United Kingdom: patients, practitioners and consultations. Lancet 2: 542–545

Harris G A 1995 Complementary therapies: their role and place within undergraduate medical education. Complementary Therapies in Medicine 3 (3): 167–170

Hockey L 1991 In: McMahon R Pearson A (eds) Nursing as therapy. Chapman and Hall, London, p x

Knape J 1998 Complementary therapies and the registered nurse, midwife and health visitor. Complementary Therapies in Nursing and Midwifery 3 (2): 54–56

Rankin-Box D 1995 Competence in the clinical setting: issues in nursing practice. Complementary Therapies in Medicine 3 (1): 25–27

Reilly D Taylor M 1993 Summary of methods and achievements. Developing integrated medicine. Complementary Therapies in Medicine 1 (supp): 6

Stone J 1999a Government plans to regulate voluntary and private healthcare. Complementary Therapies in Nursing and Midwifery 5 (6):

Stone J 1999b Using complementary therapies within nursing: some ethical and legal considerations. Complementary Therapies in Nursing and Midwifery 5 (3): 46–50

Trevelyan J 1998 Future of complementary medicine: training, status and the European perspective – Part 2. Complementary Therapies in Nursing and Midwifery 4 (4): 108–110

UKCC 1992a The Scope of Professional Practice. UKCC, London

UKCC 1992b Standards for the Administration of Medicines. UKCC, London

SECTION 1

Introducing complementary therapies in the workplace

2 Choosing a therapy

Clare Byrne

INTRODUCTION

When considering the use of a therapy two principal issues arise – the selection of a therapy for personal treatment and consideration of selection of a therapy/course in which to train. These issues are addressed separately and guidelines to facilitate selection are presented.

Under common law in the UK anyone can set up as a practitioner (or trainer); it is 'enshrined in a royal charter signed by Henry VIII' (Trevalyn 1998), and so an informed guide to the selection and use of a therapy is valuable.

In 1993, the British Medical Association (BMA) suggested that approximately 180 different therapies are practised in the UK. More recently Ernst (1996) acknowledges how complementary medicine has become big business, with a third to one-half of the general population using one or more forms of complementary therapy. To date only osteopathy has obtained legislative power to sanction individuals guilty of malpractice. For many therapies, work continues towards developing and monitoring educational standards and practice competencies. Against this background, the selection of a therapy for personal or client use can be difficult.

When choosing a therapy for oneself or for a client group it is valuable to have a wider perspective of the different therapies:

- Many complementary therapies represent systems of medicine; for example, acupuncture, homeopathy and herbalism. This is in contrast to treatments such as iridology, which is primarily a diagnostic tool, or biofeedback, massage and aromatherapy, which are primarily therapeutic (Pietroni 1990, Rankin-Box 1991).

- Some complementary therapies are derived from past cultural and social structures, such as the ancient Egyptian and Chinese civilizations. The approach taken to evaluating the effectiveness and suitability of such therapies may differ from that of orthodox scientific medical interventions. Stevensen (1992b) suggests that although the more physical, obvious and therefore measurable effects of a complementary therapy may make it easier to evaluate scientifically, the patient's response is also important.

■ Certain complementary therapies build upon the therapeutic relationship (McMahon & Pearson 1991, Wright 1995, Ersser 1997); care covers not only the physical aspects of a person's condition but also the emotional, mental, psychological and spiritual dimensions.

CHOOSING A COMPLEMENTARY THERAPY WITHIN A HEALTH CARE SETTING

The following criteria for choice of therapy were identified by Wafer (1994) when exploring the introduction of complementary therapies into a busy unit for care of the elderly:

■ The therapy could be used in everyday practice
■ The therapy would complement interdisciplinary care
■ The therapy could be realistically introduced
■ The therapy should be non-invasive
■ The therapy should provide relaxation and comfort.

Other authors such as Armstrong & Waldron (1991), Stevensen (1992a) and Burke & Sikora (1992) have also identified criteria for therapy selection in different clinical areas. Additional considerations are as follows:

■ Who is the therapy for?
■ Are research data available to substantiate the use of the therapy?
■ Is a nurse able to provide the therapy or will the therapy be provided by a specialized practitioner?
■ Is the therapy being used as part of an interdisciplinary health care team approach?
■ What is the cost and who will pay if the therapy is not available on the NHS?
■ What are the resource implications, e.g. time, space, training, materials?
■ What are the legal implications of use of the therapy, including insurance and informed consent?

CONSUMER GUIDE

In 1993, the Royal College of Nursing issued a consumer checklist (developed by the Complementary Therapies in Nursing Special Interest Group [CTINSIG]) for complementary therapies, to help patients or clients feel more confident about choosing a therapy. Some of the points they identified are listed below:

- What are the therapist's qualifications and how long was the training?
- Is the therapist a member of a recognized, registered body with codes of practice?
- Can the therapist provide the address and telephone number of this organization to check?
- Is the therapy available on the NHS?
- Can a GP delegate care to the therapist?
- Is this the most appropriate complementary therapy for the particular problem?
- Does the therapist send a letter to the GP advising of any treatment received?
- Can the patient/client claim for the therapy through a private health insurance scheme?
- Are the patient records confidential?
- What is the cost of the treatment?
- How many treatments will be needed (and therefore what is the total cost)?
- What insurance cover does the therapist have?

CHOOSING A COURSE

Carers, such as nurses, occupational therapists and physiotherapists, who have experienced the benefits of complementary therapies or who recognize their potential for enhancing their current therapeutic role often proceed to train in a therapy. In reply to constant requests from its members, the Royal College of Nursing, Department of Nursing Policy and Practice, published, in association with the CTINSIG, guidelines in 1992 called 'Choosing a complementary therapies course – what should you consider?' These guidelines are outlined here. Whilst they are concerned with nursing, they could readily be used by other health care disciplines.

First, it is important to examine personal reasons for wanting to take a complementary therapy course. These might be:

- to use such therapies in conjunction with nursing skills
- to develop a new career
- to enhance self-awareness.

Then there are the obvious practical considerations:

- what qualifications are needed
- the length of the course

- how much the course costs (remember time is a cost)
- whether an employer will help fund the course
- if there is scope for development in the nurse's current area of work.

Some useful feedback can be got from others who have undertaken a particular complementary therapies course. It is also helpful to visit the institution and speak to the trainers. (Note that correspondence courses are best avoided as they are often difficult to complete or validate.)

It is essential to determine if the course is validated by any examining bodies, whether there is accreditation, and what European Community regulations affect the therapy in question. Regarding course content and structure, check which of the following are included:

- supervised training practice
- anatomy and physiology
- practical examination
- theory examination
- supervised clinical practice
- counselling/communication and self-development skills
- support for the trainee therapist
- business skills.

Other questions to ask are:

- Does the course take an holistic approach?
- Is there support for the trainee therapist?
- What are the qualifications of the teaching staff, and are they appropriate?
- How many will be in the class (what is the tutor/pupil ratio)?

Finally, a 'taster' is a good way to get the feel of a course before making a commitment.

Rankin-Box (1998) notes how in response to demand, nurses have spearheaded the development of generic, undergraduate and post-graduate university validated courses in many aspects of complementary medicine. However, courses are no longer designed exclusively for nurses but involve multidisciplinary education. There are common core educational profiles which include modules on healing and spirituality, cross-cultural approaches to healing, shamanism, communication, counselling and the development of hospitals as healing environments.

Furthermore this process has encouraged debate throughout health care disciplines and an increasing interest by ever wider groups of doctors, nurses and lay practitioners in spearheading a change in the term 'complementary'. This is rapidly being superseded by the label 'integrative' medicine implying a coalition of allopathic and alternative systems of health care. Rankin-Box (1998) suggests that this will enable health care to move forward taking the best of both worlds with it so providing an informed, compassionate approach to healing.

CHOOSING A PRACTITIONER

GP clinics, health centres

Since 1993 it has been possible to delegate NHS client care to complementary therapists. Many General Practice (GP) fundholders now employ complementary therapists in their health care team. The GP must, according to the medical code of conduct, retain overall responsibility.

Professional registering organizations

The professional organizations for the different therapies should be able to provide a list of local registered practitioners. The British Holistic Medical Association (BHMA) holds names and addresses for these professional organizations – see also the addresses listed at the back of this book.

Summary

Choosing a complementary therapy, whether for personal use or to enhance the therapeutic role, entails thorough investigation of potential benefits. It is important to evaluate critically the research data available. Knowledge of the various therapies can be developed through information gathering and personal experience at workshops. Additionally, there are practical considerations such as availability of a registered practitioner. When considering training, availability of validated courses, the approval of all members of the team and consideration of how to evaluate the effectiveness of the complementary therapy intervention must be taken into account.

Those who have used complementary therapies for themselves and for their client group usually recommend proceeding with caution. Consider why and whether a therapy is needed for a specific client group. Critically evaluate the potential benefits or contraindications regarding the use of a therapy and objectively appraise the evidence underpinning a therapy and training programme offered.

REFERENCES

Armstrong F Waldran R 1991 A complementary strategy. Nursing Times 87: 34–35

Burke C Sikora K 1992 Cancer – the dual approach. Nursing Times 88: 62–66

Ernst E 1996 Complementary medicine – an objective appraisal. Butterworth Heinemann, London

Ersser S J 1997 Nursing as a therapeutic activity – an ethnography. Developments in Nursing and Healthcare 14: 13

McMahon R Pearson A 1991 Nursing as therapy. Chapman and Hall, London

Pietroni P 1990 The greening of medicine. Victor Gollancz, London

Rankin-Box D 1991 Proceed with caution. Nursing Times 87: 34–36

Rankin-Box D 1998 Keeping the balance – whim and wisdom. Positive Health December/January:

Stevensen C 1992a Appropriate therapies for nurses to practise. Nursing Standard 6: 51–52

Stevensen C 1992b Holistic power. Nursing Standard 88: 68–70

Trevalyn J 1998 On the continental shelf. Nursing Times 94 (26):

Wafer M 1994 Finding the formula to enhance care. Professional Nurse March: 414–417

Wright S G 1995 Bringing the heart back into nursing. Complementary Therapies in Nursing and Midwifery 1 (1): 15–20

FURTHER READING – JOURNALS

Knape J 1998 Complementary therapies and the registered nurse, midwife and health visitor. Complementary Therapies in Nursing and Midwifery 4: 54–56

Rankin-Box D (ed) 1988 Complementary health therapies. A guide for nurses and the caring professions. Croom Helm, London

Rankin-Box D 1993 Innovations in practice: complementary therapies in nursing. Complementary Therapies in Medicine 2: 27–35

Thomas R 1999 The training revolution. Journal of Alternative and Complementary Medicine. August: 27–29

3 Managing change in the workplace

Denise Rankin-Box

'There is nothing permanent except change'

Heraclitus (540–475 BC)

INTRODUCTION

There are a number of general issues associated with the introduction of complementary therapies into a clinical setting and these can be illustrated by some examples of general strategies of change. The examples provided here are not exhaustive but hopefully show how innovative approaches to health care may be implemented within the clinical setting.

When integrating complementary therapies in orthodox health care, the rate and direction of change in a particular setting can vary markedly. Some pioneers will encounter few problems, but they are perhaps in the minority. Many others will face seemingly insurmountable hurdles to changing practice or introducing a new approach. Some will identify the direction in which they wish to develop but fail to select an appropriate strategy to facilitate the change. This chapter looks at ways of easing the process of change.

CHANGE

Change is an inevitable aspect of daily life. However, as Toffler (1970) suggests, the rate of change has implications distinct from the direction of change. In the myriad organizational structures and institutions of today's society, rate and direction of change may not be well-matched. Frequently individuals or groups are exorted to take on board new ideas that have radical implications for their work. Varying rates of change across society or a profession can result in considerable stress or burnout as people attempt to adjust and adapt to unprecedented change (Moss–Kanter 1984).

In the field of health care, organizations are under pressure to cut costs and yet improve services in the face of government regulation and the growth of cost-effective and profit-oriented hospital structures (Moss–Kanter 1984). In the midst of the rapid change in many areas of health care there has been critical appraisal and reflection on the nature of nursing and the priorities and direction of health care delivery. Complementary approaches within health care represent one aspect of change that has been initiated mainly by nurses rather than management. In contrast to the seemingly impersonal organizational changes in health care, this approach gives greater priority to the needs of clients and their carers than to those of the organization. It reflects a radical change of direction in the philosophy of health care provision. Identifying the direction of change implies reflective acknowledgement that things have moved on; values have shifted and a restructuring of health care provision is required. Direction provides the vision for change. The rate at which such a change can be successfully implemented is influenced by issues associated with the management of change.

Wright (1989) suggests that nurses can be effective agents of change. Nursing can influence social and individual health and wellbeing, and Wright argues that if we believe our actions are utilitarian then there is a responsibility to ensure we control the delivery and quality of our service; this implies both individual and political commitment to change. Wright notes that because change produces individual stress related to a perceived lack of control, we must determine the nature and direction of change. A knowledge of the process of change is essential for the effective integration of complementary approaches to health care. It encourages nurses to be proactive in determining the course of the profession (Wright 1989), and to become masters not slaves of change (Moss–Kanter 1983).

APPROACHES TO CHANGE

People differ in their ability to manage change (Dobson et al 1988). Some welcome change whilst others prefer more stable conditions. The selection of a particular model should take into account the situation, beliefs, values and behaviour of the people who are to experience the change (Haffer 1986).

There are a number of models of change theory in the literature, such as Lewin (1953), Seifert & Clinebell (1969), Lippitt (1970). They highlight ways in which change may occur:

- Lewin (1953) suggests three phases – unfreezing, moving and then refreezing – a process by which an individual is encouraged to reflect critically upon current practice, new concepts are introduced and considered and finally the idea is adopted and change occurs creating another status quo.
- Seifert & Clinebell (1969) and Lippitt (1970) adopt a problem-solving approach to the management of change involving

diagnosis of a problem and subsequent steps taken to manage the process of change effectively.

The approach adopted depends on the environment in which the change is to be introduced. The steps listed here provide a general guide and build upon the stages identified by Lippitt (1970).

- Recognize the need for change
- Diagnose why
- Team recognizes why
- Team recognizes the need for change
- Identify the aim
- Consider alternate courses of action/practice
- Set clear, achievable objectives
- Reinforce positively when objectives are met by the team
- Monitor and evaluate the process of change
- Review and appraise.

STRATEGIES FOR CHANGE

There are three key strategies for change: power coercive, rational empirical and normative re-educative.

Power coercive. This assumes a 'top-down' approach to change. Underpinning the strategy is a belief that knowledge is power which can be used to achieve a desired outcome (Keyzer 1989). It is commonly associated with hierarchical systems of management.

Rational empirical. This assumes people are rational and self-interested and will view change positively, as long as there are benefits (Bennis et al 1976). An example of the rational empirical approach is telling people that cigarette smoking is dangerous to health in order to alter smoking behaviour.

Normative re-educative. This is influenced by the perception a group or individual has of both the need for and value of change. Keyzer (1989) notes that this approach offers a means of drawing upon the organization's perceptions of the need for change as well as individual or group needs. It requires team participation in change and forms the basis for the belief that the process of change should build upon collaboration between the client and the agent of change.

A normative re-educative strategy is commonly considered the most effective stance to adopt for change. It facilitates a multidisciplinary approach to changing health care by the introduction of a complementary therapy.

KEY ISSUES TO BE AWARE OF WHEN MANAGING CHANGE

The introduction of an innovative approach to health care must be carefully planned before implementation. Where possible, a normative re-educative strategy will facilitate a multidisciplinary approach towards the introduction of a therapy within daily practice. Some common considerations for the introduction of complementary therapies in the work setting are listed next (adapted from Moss–Kanter 1984 – an account of hurdles encountered when attempting to manage change). They reflect concerns raised by many nurse practitioners attempting to introduce complementary therapies and holistic procedures to daily practice.

- **Loss of control**

  Attitudes to change are influenced by the extent to which people feel in control. Lack of control makes people feel powerless. Moss–Kanter (1984) suggests 'it is powerlessness that corrupts – not power'. Individuals not in control may seek to undermine the process of change.

  Solution: Offer people choices and a sense of ownership over the change/selection of a therapy.

- **Excess uncertainty**

  Individuals resist change if they are not sure where the change will take them and what the long-term implications are.

  Solution: Divide any large-scale or radical change into small achievable steps to reduce the sense of risk or threat. Giving frequent information and updates can allay anxieties as well as providing a clear vision of overall change.

- **Innovative therapies are different**

  Rapid change can be exhausting because habits and rituals are upturned or removed. Learning new routines and patterns of care may make people feel they no longer know how to do their work – and this can be both stressful and draining.

  Solution: Highlight the similarities between previous, familiar practices and new therapies. For instance, preparing a client for a massage, reflexology or aromatherapy treatment has similarities with, for example, preparation for blanket bathing, pressure care or other forms of physical care. By highlighting the familiar, the team are able to retain some habits and routines.

- **Losing face**

  In the enthusiasm of introducing something you are convinced is a better approach to nursing care, there is a danger that past actions may be perceived as 'not good enough' or 'wrong'.

Solution: Put past actions into context. Previous actions may have been excellent. However, times have changed and information and practices not readily available before may now be considered as potential ways in which to improve already high standards of care.

■ **Change is work**
Introducing change to the clinical setting takes considerable work. There is the inception and analysis of an idea, strategic planning, discussion, the process of implementation and finally evaluation of effectiveness.
Solution: Acknowledge this with the team. Be honest. Where possible, reward hard work to facilitate commitment to the change.

A crucial aspect of successful change is effective communication amongst the multidisciplinary team. When attempting to introduce complementary therapies into the clinical environment it is essential that anxieties and concerns as well as hopes and enthusiasm for new practices be openly shared and discussed.

CHANGE AND COMPLEMENTARY THERAPIES

Whilst movement towards the integration of complementary therapies in daily health care and NHS practice appears slow, increasing attention is being afforded to education and training, regulation and research and development (FIM 1997). Therapies are being perceived as part of a movement towards *integrated medicine*, a term unheard of only a few years ago.

In the UK approximately 4–5 million people a year now consult complementary practitioners and in the US an estimated $15 billion per annum is spent on complementary therapies (Eisenberg et al 1993, Stone 1999).

In 1997, the Foundation for Integrated Medicine (FIM) produced a key report in the field of CAM entitled, 'Integrated healthcare: a way forward for the next five years'. The report highlighted four key areas to be addressed in forthcoming years – research and development; education and training; regulation and delivery mechanisms. The UK does not currently operate a centralized commission overseeing the training and practice of complementary therapies, preferring, for the moment at least, to leave regulation and training in specific therapies to the relevant organizational bodies. However, it will be interesting to monitor future developments in this field and there are considerable efforts underway to develop and promote open and collegiate dialogue across the field of complementary medicine.

It will take time for each of the stages of change management to take place – not least because various therapy organizations are at varying stages of the change process. In this respect open communication and team work are essential.

Summary

The introduction of complementary therapies into current nursing practice carries with it many unique challenges and opportunities. It is, however, inextricably linked with the management of change. How an individual or group chooses to approach the process of change will influence the extent to which an innovative aspect of nursing care is accepted by the team as part of mainstream care.

Managing the introduction of complementary health care within orthodox nursing will, if strategically planned, take time. Many issues such as research, establishing safety and efficacy of therapies, policy development and standard setting, should form part of the process of change before therapies are practised in the clinical environment.

A knowledge of the process of change empowers and enables nurses proactively to manage and shape future nursing practice.

REFERENCES

Bennis W G Benne K D Chin R Corey K E 1976 The planning of change. Holt Rinehart & Winston, London

Dobson C B Hardy M Heyes S Humphreys A Humphreys P 1988 Understanding psychology. Weidenfeld & Nicholson, London

Eisenberg et al 1993 Unconventional medicine in the United States. Prevalence, costs and patterns of use. New England Journal of Medicine 328: 246–252

FIM 1997 Integrated healthcare: a way forward for the next five years? FIM, London

Haffer A 1986 Facilitating change. Nursing Administration 16: 18–22

Keyzer D 1989 Meeting the challenge: strategies for implementing change. In: Wright S G (ed) Changing nursing practice. Edward Arnold, London

Lewin K 1953 Research studies in group decisions. Evanston, Row Peterson. Cited by: Brooten D A 1984 Managerial leadership in nursing. Lippincott, Philadelphia

Lippitt G 1970 Visualizing change: model building and the change process. New York Association. Cited by Brooten D A 1984 Managerial leadership in nursing. Lippincott, Philadelphia

Moss-Kanter R 1983 The change masters. Routledge, New York

Moss-Kanter R 1984 Managing the human side of change. AMACOM A Division of American Management Association. Reprinted from: Management Review April 1985: 52–56

Seifert H Clinebell H 1969 Personal growth and social change. Westminster, Philadelphia. Cited by: Brooten D A 1984 Managerial leadership in nursing. Lippincott, Philadelphia

Stone J 1999 Using complementary therapies within nursing: some ethical and legal considerations. Complementary Therapies in Nursing and Midwifery 5 (3): 46–50

Toffler A 1970 Future shock. Pan, London

Wright S G (ed) 1989 Changing nursing practice. Edward Arnold, London

4 Policy development

Denise Rankin-Box   Maxine McVey

INTRODUCTION

To date there are few national guidelines determining the practice of complementary therapies. However, paragraph 39 of the UKCC Standards for the Administration of Medicines states that the practice of complementary therapies should be based upon sound principles, available knowledge and skill (UKCC 1992c). An increasing number of regional health authorities have developed policy statements and guidelines that stipulate forms and standards of practice (Bath 1991, West Berkshire 1992, St Bartholomew's 1993). This chapter examines a range of issues in policy development and the successful implementation of complementary therapies within clinical practice. Policy development currently falls within the remit of a working party established to address a range of issues associated with complementary therapies in the clinical setting. The establishment of a working party, its aims and subsequent policy development are also discussed here.

A POLICY

A policy is a constitution, a course of action, a principle adapted or proposed by government party, business or an individual and is a set of guidelines sanctioned by those in authority, whether members of the Trust board in a self-governed hospital or Members of Parliament. It states the intentions in a given situation, and guides good conduct in practical situations. Policy documents are commonly likened to codes of conduct or practices that define or establish principles and standards of practice.

RATIONALE FOR POLICY DEVELOPMENT IN COMPLEMENTARY THERAPIES

There are a number of reasons why a policy should be developed for the integration of complementary therapies into clinical practice. All qualified nurses are bound by the UKCC Code of Professional Conduct (1992a), and Guidelines for Professional Practice

(UKCC 1996) accountability is an integral part of this code. It is generally within the practical sphere that a nurse practitioner has to make judgements and be answerable for them. Policy documents usually state intentions in a given situation, with the aim of having the guidelines sanctioned by those in authority. As a rule, issues are addressed and where possible, solutions proposed. A policy further seeks to safeguard the safety of the patient and public.

In conjunction with the UKCC Guidelines of Professional Practice (1996) policy development in complementary therapies assists nurses towards identifying competent practice. In this respect, a policy promotes and classifies principles of practice directed at safeguarding the patient and the public. Additionally, policy development serves to reinforce the UKCC guidelines by highlighting issues associated with professional accountability within practice. A final consideration is the establishment of clear definitions and measurable criteria upon which clinical practice in this field can be evaluated. This latter aspect is important since it is the issue which will assist in determining efficiency of treatments.

NATIONAL POLICY DEVELOPMENT

In 1997 the Foundation for Integrated Medicine (FIM) produced a report addressing a range of key issues associated with the integration of complementary therapies within current health care practice. The report notes that, in general, policy will determine what is included in public sector provision and debate about need will depend on how need is defined. How a national framework will be developed will depend on how information and resources are managed, assessment of quality of care and appropriate measures of quality of life and health gain (FIM 1997).

SETTING UP A WORKING PARTY FOR COMPLEMENTARY THERAPIES

The team selected for policy development should be multidisciplinary. The members of the group are required to have a commitment to the aims of the working party, with each individual having a role to play to ensure the successful implementation of complementary therapies within the clinical setting. The team structure might be as follows:

- Membership/Trust manager – to provide information relating to cost and management issues
- Nurses who have an interest/qualification in complementary therapies – to have an understanding of the code of professional

conduct; knowledge of the therapies – to evaluate practical issues related to their integration and implementation

- Health care professionals from different clinical areas – knowledge of different specialties to establish whether or not the policy is relevant to the nurses using it in a range of settings
- Multidisciplinary team, e.g. doctors, physiotherapists, pharmacists – to ensure collaboration between disciplines
- Links with other health policy initiatives and Department of Health developments towards research-based practice
- If possible a person with experience of policy development – to facilitate policy development and assist in developing a framework defining the aims, objectives and issues relating to the formulation of a policy.

When meetings involve more than ten people, individual participation becomes difficult (Dobree 1991); initial teams of about five to seven members are recommended. Some members may only be required to attend a meeting when items relevant to their positions are discussed. Questions for initial consideration include:

- By whose authority is the group established?
- Is the group just to develop a policy?
- Is there a responsibility to establish how many nurses are practising complementary therapies in the hospital/region?
- Does the group have a role in encouraging and enabling therapies to be practised?
- Resource implications for facilitating committee meetings.

Organization of the team

In addition to team selection, the organization of the team should be addressed at initial meetings to set the framework for future decisions.

- Role of chairperson – the selection and the definition of the responsibilities as link person for communication within the group
- Secretarial support – the necessary skills to be able to fulfil the position, for example typing, recording minutes and administrative duties
- Venue of meetings – if possible an identified place, away from distractions, e.g. clinical area
- Frequency of meetings – to maintain momentum and enable reflection and action between the meetings

- Timescale to produce a policy – objectives should be set, to be met before each meeting as well as an overall timescale for the development of a policy
- The remit of the group – additional roles identified; vice chair, remit of individuals.

The purpose of the group, its aims and objectives should be decided at the first meeting. This will guide the planning of the meetings and the activities of members and dictate when the project has been achieved.

Preliminary issues

In defining the remit and structure of the team, it will be necessary to identify the aims and objectives of the group. These may range from a defined focus on policy development to a broader remit whereby the group acts as a hospital or regional resource for matters relating to complementary therapies. The list below includes features attributable to professional practice and policy committees.

- Policy development for the use of complementary therapies
- Act as a resource for all nurses and health care professionals interested in complementary therapies
- Provide a forum for sharing and updating information in this field
- Clarify and establish organizational resources to support the development of complementary therapies.

Any policy development requires the establishment of baseline knowledge in order to define its remit. Methods of acquiring this include:

- Reviewing existing health authority policies on complementary therapies – identifying key issues to be addressed
- Conducting a literature search to appraise critically the substantive base upon which a therapy is established and therapeutic claims affirmed
- Organizing a survey to identify consumer demand for specific therapies within a hospital or region
- Establishing the current usage of specific therapies within nursing practice and identifying competent practitioners.

This list is a general guide and not exhaustive: the field is rapidly developing and therefore certain issues take on greater or lesser importance depending upon current social and political factors. It can be valuable to define clear terms of reference and in particular, links should be established with existing committees.

FACTORS TO CONSIDER WHEN FORMULATING A POLICY

Some areas commonly included in current policies addressing complementary therapies are as follows:

- Title of policy
- Identification of aim – overall goal
- Definition of terms used within the policy
- Identification of objectives – attainable goals that can be evaluated and measured
- Identification and evaluation of research studies on therapeutic efficacy and any treatment claims made
- Identification and critical evaluation of established training courses
- Identification of established organizations with recognized educational criteria in particular therapies
- Human resource issues – management
- Identification of educational criteria to determine competent practitioners within the hospital/health care region
- Definition of competency to practise
- Identification of existing registers of practitioners and criteria for inclusion on the register
- Evaluation of existing health policies in this field
- Establishment of links and possible inclusion of an experienced member of a previous policy development team on the proposed team
- Establishment of links with other organizations involved in development of complementary therapies within health care (e.g. the RCN Complementary Therapies in Nursing Forum)
- Identification of therapies/techniques to be included
- Definitions of and information about therapies
- Contraindications for use of certain therapies
- Professional bodies who may facilitate training and integration of a therapy in to the health care setting
- Development of a multidisciplinary team approach towards the use of therapies in the health care setting
- Evaluation of a therapy
- Financial considerations – cost-effectiveness of a therapy
- Ongoing research considerations
- Links between various regional policies

- Defining organizational responsibilities
- Identification of policy standards in line with national and European legislature
- Informed consent
- Insurance
- Documentation.

Key issues

The key issues listed here are central to policy development. They are influenced by the clinical environment and the therapeutic modality to be used and some may be explored or defined in more detail according to the needs of specific clinical centres:

- Professional autonomy
- Accountability and responsibility
- Competency to practise
- Consent
- Consultation and collaboration
- General management issues
- Documentation
- Insurance
- Ethico-legal issues (see chapter 7).

Accountability and responsibility

Accountability is inextricably linked with terms such as liability and responsibility (see chapter 7). Many nurses interpret accountability and responsibility as being synonymous. This is understandable since the terms are frequently used interchangeably. Accountability originates from responsibility (Pearson & Vaughan 1990). Gardener (1992) states that accountability is dependent on knowledge, competence and experience. As knowledge and experience increase, competencies are more formally established. Some questions related to accountability in the use of complementary therapies and policy development are as follows:

- Are there specific issues to be addressed with specific therapies?
- What are the legal parameters of practice?
- Are those responsible for an area, accountable for that area?
- Are accountability and responsibility the same issue?
- Can a therapist be responsible and not accountable?
- Is accountability mandatory or a choice for the qualified nurse?

- What are the implications for accountability in relation to complementary therapies?

Stone (1999) has described a number of key issues associated with ethical and legal considerations in the field.

Lewis & Bate (1982) suggest accountability refers to 'formal obligation to disclose'. Thus, as a therapist you should be able to state:

- What it is you are trying to achieve – defining the goal in selecting and using a complementary therapy
- How you are trying to achieve it – selecting an action, the procedure involved in a therapy
- Why you are trying to achieve it – developing a knowledge base, being aware of and able critically to appraise the substantive research base underlying selected therapies
- The outcome of your actions – your evaluation, the development of an evaluation procedure for both the client and therapist.

As a nurse you must be able to give explanations for your actions and conduct, to answer as the one responsible (UKCC Guidelines for Professional Practice 1996). Binnie et al (1984) list three kinds of accountability:

- To the client or patient – a patient has the right to expect a service that maintains a high standard of care
- To the profession and the public throughout the UKCC – this is expressed in the Code of Professional Conduct (UKCC 1992a)
- To colleagues – most job descriptions contain a clause regarding the person(s) to whom nurses are accountable.

Accountability is often regarded as having to answer for an action when something goes wrong. It is actually more complex and is linked to evaluation, and how professional performance is monitored. Thus a critical appraisal of intended actions and the implications of those actions in their entirety should also be addressed. The implications of complementary therapies should be carefully thought through before practice and nurses should evaluate whether they feel competent to practise (UKCC 1996).

Competency to practise

The Guidelines for Professional Practice (UKCC 1996) state that: 'it is vitally important that you ensure that the introduction of any of these therapies is always in the best interests and safety of the patients and clients'.

Being accountable is to some extent dependent upon having the authority and autonomy to act but this may not always occur. This relates to the nurse and manager agreeing to the use of the organization's resources. It is suggested that in complementary therapies authorization is directly linked with competency to practise in association with the development of a multidisciplinary team approach within the clinical setting and across the therapeutic specialism. It is necessary that each individual nurse recognizes personal competency skills and that these can be evaluated to ensure the client is safeguarded. Considerations may include:

- Safeguarding the patient/client
- Ensuring practice is within the UKCC guidelines
- Recognizing limits to competency – not exceeding personal skills
- Defining criteria for a competent educational programme
- Recognizing contraindications to treatments
- Working within a multidisciplinary team – not countermanding medical instructions
- Promoting the safe and effective use of complementary therapies
- Demonstrating the ability to perform therapeutic techniques that can be evaluated and which meet established educational criteria.

Whilst many complementary therapies are frequently presented as an expansion of the nurse's role, certain therapies make definitive therapeutic and treatment claims. Some therapies claim diagnostic and treatment processes analogous to medicine, e.g. herbalism, acupuncture and to some extent aromatherapy. Where there is the potential for interaction with conventional medical treatment, collaborative multidisciplinary approaches to practice are needed. The General Medical Council guidelines for doctors, 'Professional Conduct and Discipline. Fitness to Practise' (GMC 1992), sets out conditions for the delegation of medical duties to nurses and others; paragraphs 42 and 43 of this document state that doctors who delegate treatment or other pro-cedures must ensure the person to whom they are delegated is competent to carry them out. It is, however, also appropriate to consider developing the nurse's role as a practitioner of complementary therapy independently of medically delegated duties.

Who is competent to practise? Answering this question may be fundamental to the aims of the group and affects the key issues formulating the criteria for the policy. Candidates include:

- Qualified staff with a recognized course
- A qualified nurse who has received instruction in a therapy and is under the supervision of the qualified staff with a recognized course

- A student or a care assistant
- A therapist who is not a nurse.

Competency through education. The patient/client is ethically protected by the UKCC and the nurse's professional responsibility. To help nurses considering a complementary therapy, guidelines have been formulated by the RCN, Department of Nursing Policy and Practice, Complementary Therapies in Nursing Special Interest Group (see Chapter 2 on Choosing a therapy). The significant aspects of training are:

- desirable course contents
- a period of supervision
- formal examination which enables a person to obtain insurance.

Stone (1999) also discusses the issue of competency to practise, and issues surrounding regulation, research education and delivery mechanisms are detailed in the report by the Foundation for Integrated Medicine entitled 'Integrated healthcare: a way forward for the next five years?' (FIM 1997)

Consent

It is essential that policy documents address the issue of informed consent. Informed consent requires that the patient receives sufficient information to take a decision about the therapy and implies that the person giving the information has a sound knowledge base. If a nurse has insufficient information, clients should be referred to additional sources. Informed consent should be obtained before practice, with the client receiving information about the therapy detailing benefits, contraindications and side-effects. The main areas for policy consideration are as follows:

- Should consent be documented?
- What form should be used?
- What are the legal implications of developing a form?
- Can a formal consent form be completed by a therapist who is not a nurse?

Consultation and collaboration

When developing innovative clinical practice it is valuable to ensure multidisciplinary collaboration. This is linked to competency to practise and the safety of the clients. Questions for consideration include:

- How can this be achieved?
- Do specific therapies limit which patients/clients can be treated?

- Should the consultation be documented?
- What happens if a patient wishes to have a therapy and the medical practitioner is not in favour?
- What if the patient was using a therapy prior to being in the care of a medical practitioner?

The policy may not be able to answer all these questions; some issues will need to be resolved locally and not by policy.

General management issues

The effectiveness of the therapy needs to be considered from a managerial and human resources perspective. For example:

- Does the manager have a responsibility to ensure a nurse has credentials to practise?
- Can the manager justify the use of the organization's resources?
- Is a therapy cost-effective?
- Are there cost implications in relation to staff training?
- Is there a case for a clinical specialist – who may not be a nurse?
- What are the purchaser's/patient's views on complementary therapies?
- Are there financial means to conduct studies to determine cost efficiency and effectiveness of a therapy within health care and establish resources for a therapy?

Documentation

It is important to record the complementary therapy treatment in the patient's care plan and to evaluate its effectiveness. There is uncertainty about the true benefits of many therapies over and above the well-recognized 'placebo' response to therapy given by a committed carer. Therefore it is an integral aspect of professional nursing to document and evaluate each treatment. Nurses should be prepared to undertake more research into complementary therapies to enhance the credibility of their practice.

Insurance

It is advisable that a therapist has his/her own public liability insurance. A recognized course should enable the therapist to obtain this. The types of therapies that can be covered in the policy may be dictated by an indemnity insurance via a trade union or professional body. The RCN provides a list of therapies currently identified and covered by professional indemnity insurance. Additionally the health authority may wish to provide further cover. Check with the legal department of the health authority for guidelines.

Summary

The implementation of certain therapies within clinical practice is dependent on nurses taking the initiative and expanding their scope of practice. In incorporating therapies within nursing practice it is hoped that a more holistic approach to care can be achieved.

REFERENCES

Binnie A et al 1984 A systematic approach to nursing care. Open University Press, Milton Keynes

Complementary Therapies in Nursing Special Interest Group 1993 Choosing a complementary therapies course. RCN, London

Dobree L 1991 The meeting game. Nursing Standard 6: 45–47

FIM 1997 Integrated healthcare: a way forward for the next five years? FIM, London

Gardner J H 1992 Where the buck stops. Nursing 5:

GMC 1992 Professional Conduct and Discipline. Fitness to Practice, para. 42

Lewis F M Bate M V 1982 Clarifying autonomy and accountability to nursing service – part 11. Journal of Nursing Administration

Pearson A Vaughan B 1990 Nursing models for practice. Heinemann Nursing, Oxford, p 49

Stone J 1999 Using complementary therapies within nursing: some ethical and legal considerations. Complementary Therapies in Nursing and Midwifery 5 (3): 46–50

UKCC 1992a Code of Professional Conduct, 3rd edn. UKCC, London

UKCC 1992b Scope of Professional Practice. UKCC, London

UKCC 1992c Standards for the Administration of Medicines. UKCC, London

UKCC 1996 Guidelines for Professional Practice. UKCC London

FURTHER READING – JOURNALS

Armstrong F Waldren R 1991 A complementary strategy. Nursing Times 87: 34–35

Burke C Kikora K 1992 Cancer – the dual approach. Nursing Times 88: 62–66

Crowther D 1991 Complementary therapy in practice. Nursing Standard 5: 25–27

Rankin-Box D 1991 Proceed with caution. Nursing Times 87: 34–36

Stevensen C 1992 Holistic power. Nursing Times 88: 68–70

UKCC 1992 Code of Professional Conduct, 3rd edn. UKCC, London

UKCC 1992 Standards For The Administration of Medicines. UKCC Section 39, London

UKCC 1992 The Scope of Professional Practice. UKCC, London

FURTHER READING – BOOKS

BMA 1993 Complementary medicine: new approaches to good practice. British Medical Association/Oxford University Press, Oxford

Buckman R Sabbagh K 1993 Magic or medicine? An investigation into healing. Macmillan, London

Complementary therapy. London Nursing Times/Macmillan, 1993

Grant B 1993 Alternative health: A–Z of natural healthcare. Optima, London

Inglis B 1979 Natural medicine. Collins, London

Olsen K 1991 The encylopaedia of alternative health care. Piatkus, London

Rankin-Box D (ed) 1988 Complementary health therapies: a guide for nurses and the caring professions. Chapman and Hall, London

Stanway A (ed) 1987 The natural family doctor. Gaia, London

USEFUL ADDRESSES

British Holistic Medical Association
179 Gloucester Place
London NW1 6DX
Tel: 020 7262 5299

RCN Complementary Therapies in Nursing Forum
Royal College of Nursing
20 Cavendish Square
London W1M 0AB
Tel: 020 7409 333

Research Council for Complementary Medicine
505 Riverbank House
1 Putney Bridge Approach
London SW6 3JD UK
Tel: 020 7384 1772
Fax: 020 7384 1736

Institute of Complementary Medicine
PO Box 194
London SE16 1QZ

Foundation for Integrated Medicine
International House
59 Compton Road
London N1 2YT
Tel: 020 7688 1881
Fax: 020 7688 1882

Health Authorities that have produced policies on complementary therapies

West Berkshire Health Authority 1992
Royal Berks & Battle Hospital Trust
Royal Berkshire Hospital
Craven Road
Reading RG1 5AN

Bath District Health Authority 1989
Royal United Hospital
Combe Park Bath
Avon BA1 3NG

With thanks to the above Health Authorities who have given their permission to act as policy resources for people interested in developing policies in the field.

5 Clinical supervision

Peter A Mackereth

INTRODUCTION

The rising interest by nurses in complementary therapies signalled by the demand for educational programmes and texts such as this clearly demonstrates an awakening to the healing potential of nurses and nursing. While there are many forms of alternative and complementary therapies, a commonly shared belief is that both the therapist and the intervention work together to help people heal themselves. An emphasis on the relationship and the individuality of the patient requires practitioners to be alive to their work and the moment. Thoughtful reflection and sensitive application of skills can facilitate this. More than this it requires cultivating a way of being with another sustained by learning about how we relate to others and understand ourselves. As early as 1994 the author recommended that nurses using or intending to integrate complementary therapies into their nursing practice consider engaging in clinical supervision (Mackereth & Gale 1994). More recently Cromwell et al (1999) report that monthly clinical supervision sessions were used to support practitioners offering a pilot reflexology and massage service in a ward area. This chapter introduces the reader to the concept of clinical supervision and explores issues related to complementary therapies.

RATIONALE FOR CLINICAL SUPERVISION

Fundamental to clinical supervision is the provision of time, space and a supportive relationship that enables practitioners to reflect on their own practice and professional development. Supervision will also be open to professional and organizational differences, so it is essential to clarify its purpose. Faugier & Butterworth (1994) have described clinical supervision as an 'exchange between practising professionals to enable the development of professional skills'. The practice of therapists participating in supervision originates in the development of psychoanalysis (Butterworth & Faugier 1992). This forms an essential part of the training and ongoing practice of psychotherapy and counselling. Psychotherapy supervision for example provides a space for analysis of the therapist's work, including the exploration of transference and countertransference issues. It is important to acknowledge that psychotherapists and counsellors engage in personal therapy as an essential part of their training and post-registration support. Personal growth has also been claimed as potential outcome of clinical supervision for nurses (Butterworth & Faugier 1992, McCallion & Baxter 1995a, Jones 1996). Yegdich (1998) is critical of the wholesale acceptance in nursing of personal growth through supervision, suggesting that the intimate therapeutic work with the patient might be lost in favour of focusing on the nurse. The supervisor is clearly not the supervisee's therapist, but they may use their skills to guide and support an individual in exploring how they might pursue personal development. For example a bereavement issue affecting the author's work required exploration and support both in supervision and psychotherapy (Mackereth 1998). Typically supervision time can be spent in exploring issues arising from working with patients and possibly also managing an NHS complementary therapy clinic, as well as refining interpersonal and complementary therapy skills. Separating personal growth and professional development issues can be complex and requires careful analysis and reflection so that supervision does not become personal therapy for the supervisee. Engaging in the debate, having clear supervision contracts and supervision for supervisors can all contribute towards clarifying the boundaries of this work.

CLINICAL SUPERVISION IN NURSING AND COMPLEMENTARY THERAPIES

Incidents alerting the public to concerns about poor and even dangerous practice have been part of a drive to introduce and promote clinical supervision, the highest profile being the Beverley Allitt case (Allitt Inquiry 1994). This association to preventing harm is in sharp contrast to Jones's (1995) view that supervision needs to be seen as helping nurses to 'attain excellence' in clinical practice and 'fulfill their professional potential' (Jones 1995, p 212). Evidence to support clinical supervision in nursing, and more specifically for those working with complementary therapies, is currently largely anecdotal or derived from a small number of studies. Benefits for nurses and the service include confidence-building, avoidance of burnout (Hallberg et al 1994), improved staff morale and job satisfaction with implications for retention of staff and reducing sickness/absences (Butterworth et al 1996). An evaluation of a 23-site study providing clinical supervision for 18 months reported that nurses had welcomed the activity in providing a space to reflect and be supported in managing work that can be harrowing, challenging and upsetting (White et al 1998). Aside from supervision relationships taking time to establish and evaluate, it is not readily available to the majority of nurses despite support from the Department of Health and the UKCC (DoH 1993, UKCC 1995). Cutcliffe & Proctor (1998) argue that if student nurses receive training as supervisees this will help supervision move forward by facilitating their reflective and interpersonal skills, and in turn create a 'greater equality and intentionality in the working alliance' (Cutcliffe & Proctor 1998, p 346). Bishop (1994) argues that supervision not only has the potential to develop a collegiate culture but also support innovation and the sharing of research and up-to-date practice. Typically nurses who use complementary therapies are striving to provide quality care for people experiencing chronic health problems, life-threatening and life-limiting diseases (Rankin-Box 1997). In these circumstances opportunities for support and guidance may be hard to obtain. Nurses providing complementary therapies could argue that supervision is an essential component of their scope of practice (UKCC 1992). Tingle (1995) has suggested that from a legal perspective clinical supervision could operate as a 'clinical risk management tool' reducing complaints and litigation (Tingle 1995, p 794). Being proactive in seeking and organizing supervision, in consultation with a line manager, may also help to reassure patients and colleagues that accountability and quality enhancement will be paramount to the provision of complementary therapies. To see supervision as just about providing support, advice and ongoing training belittles its potential to assist the practitioner in developing a deeper understanding of both the therapy and the therapeutic relationship. Engaging regularly in reflective practice in the space provided by supervision can also help the practitioner to take the process into everyday practice, that is fine-tuning abilities to 'reflect in' practice by developing and nurturing the 'internal supervisor'. For many practitioners this inner voice often takes the position of what Jennings calls the 'harsh critic or judge' (Jennings 1999, p 65) rather than the benevolent supporter and motivator.

ORGANIZATIONAL ARRANGEMENTS

While recommending the activity of clinical supervision the UKCC has been non-prescriptive concerning its development in general nursing practice (UKCC 1995). This stance may highlight the diversity and complexities of the culture that exists in a variety of practice settings (Pritchard 1997). However, some practitioners are either waiting for it to be imposed by their managers or simply doing it for themselves. This raises questions of competency. Some organizations are being proactive by working together with clinical staff to explore a model of clinical supervision (Cromwell et al 1999). For instance supervision arrangements and requirements are now being included as part of

Box 6.1 Clinical supervision contract

Shared responsibilities for:

- Agreeing the venue, dates and times for supervision
- Avoiding rescheduling sessions where possible (ideally 24 hour notice)
- The maintenance of confidentiality within limits*
- Regularly reviewing the usefulness of the supervision
- Giving two sessions notice if discontinuing/changing supervision arrangements
- Negotiating and clarifying the focus of the supervision work at each session.

* Limits of confidentiality include acts/intentions that are illegal, break the participants' code of conduct or infringe their employment-related disciplinary policies.

complementary therapy protocols (Neil Cliffe Cancer Care Centre 1998). Although policies and protocols give guidelines for acceptable standards of practice they may not answer specific questions (McVey 1996), provide much needed support or assist the practitioner to reflect.

STRUCTURING CLINICAL SUPERVISION

To initiate supervision a contract is first formulated to provide guidance and ground rules for the work. This will usually include agreed statements concerning individual and shared responsibilities (Box 6.1).

Since supervision is concerned with the supervisee's practice and, indirectly, patient care, they must feel able to make as much use of the time and relationship as possible. Preparation and guidance by the supervisor is essential. This is further assisted by the supervisor themselves being in supervision not only for their practice, but also their supervision work. It is important to stress that preparation of supervisor alone might give a signal that it is a one-way process. Working in isolation is the antithesis of supervision. As supervisory relationships take time to develop it is important to include ongoing evaluation with a formal review at least twice a year. Clinical supervision to grow as a professional and accessible activity also requires supervisees to consider their future potential to become supervisors. This includes assessing further training and education requirements and ongoing supervision in developing their skills. Suggested steps to getting clinical supervision started are summarized in Box 6.2.

Box 6.2 Getting started with clinical supervision

- Start by gathering information about clinical supervision
- Network with other complementary therapists involved in clinical supervision
- Identify a supervisor/supervisory arrangement that best meets your needs
- Check that supervisor is also receiving supervision
- Provide and discuss proposed supervision contract, costs and supervisor/supervisory arrangement with line manager
- Initiate the activity and agree review dates and means of recording supervision sessions
- Actively engage in the process of supervision with a view to it being

Box 6.3 Clinical supervision methods/arrangements

1. Individual, with supervisor being of the same profession
2. Individual, with the supervisor being of a different profession but having shared professional focus
3. One to one peer 'co-supervision' where the individuals are of similar experience and skill
4. Group supervision with a supervisor (either as in 1 or 2 above)
5. Peer group with members sharing/contributing to facilitation/support
6. Triad supervision where a supervisor also has their own supervisor present. This is particularly helpful in teaching/developing supervisor and supervisee skills.

The most common supervision arrangements are one-to-one sessions with a supervisor lasting between 45 and 60 minutes and occurring fortnightly or monthly. Too long an interval between sessions might lead to a supervisee brooding over issues or result in participants spending the time catching up and reconnecting rather than focusing on the work (Johns 1993). There are alternative arrangements or methods of supervision (Box 6.3); each may have advantages and disadvantages. For example, Rodriguez & Goorapah (1998) believe that peer supervision could be very supportive, while McCallion & Baxter (1995b) suggest that it might perpetuate current rather than innovative practice.

SPECIFIC ISSUES FOR COMPLEMENTARY THERAPIES

Unlike mentoring and preceptorship, supervision is largely concerned with ongoing practice rather than its initiation or assessment of competence. Neither does the supervisor have to be an expert in all aspects of the supervisee's practice. This opens the door for nurses using complementary therapies to consider supervision with other health care practitioners and therapists whose experience and expertise is in complementary therapies. Such arrangements can provide opportunities for shared learning and a broadening of professional experience, but will need to be fully discussed with all parties concerned, particularly if a line manager is providing funding and/or time.

Nurses who offer complementary therapies to patients often report that they experience greater levels of attachment. The time together, coupled with the use of touch, can provide a space within which patients have been known to express fears, sadness, worries and concerns (Vickers 1996, Penson 1998, Cromwell et al 1999). Witnessing a patient crying or expressing a deep-seated anxiety requires us to think about the original therapeutic contract made with the patient at the beginning of the session. Reflexology or aromatherapy may have been offered with the aim of helping a patient to sleep, ease pain or simply relax. This very different outcome might call for gentle and sensitive containment such as sitting with the patient quietly, with their permission, until they feel ready to discuss what they need. It might be that your presence is enough or that they would like more help with their feelings. Counselling might be an option, but this requires a clear contract, time, support and the skills for that work rather than tagging it unprepared onto a complementary therapy intervention. Touch can be powerful not just for the receiver. What happens when a patient triggers feelings of fondness, discomfort or irritation? We can try to ignore it or even limit our contact with the individual or we could attempt to examine and understand the response. Supervision could provide an ideal space to discuss and make sense of these very individual and challenging situations and responses.

Supervision is not only about problems and challenges but it can provide a space in which we can receive feedback about our strengths (Hallberg et al 1994). To really hear and utilize feedback, engagement is essential to the relationship. Being open to support and praise can contribute to feeling 'potent' as a nurse and/or complementary therapist (Mackereth 1997). Engagement not only requires the supervisee to bring practice and development issues to supervision but also to participate in the analysis of their own work. The engagement is then sustained and deepened by maintaining effective dialogue between the supervisee and supervisor, including appraisal and evaluation of their work together.

Summary

For the author supervision has been an important and developmental cornerstone to the safety and potency of complementary therapy practice (Mackereth 1997). In considering the shift from doing 'trained' complementary work to 'being' a therapist, Westland believes that supervision can enable practitioners to learn to be 'not knowing and all that that entails' (Westland 1993, p 5). This spaciousness in the process is dependent on commitment and engagement, effective dialogue and clear understanding of the supervision contract. In return supervision offers a space that can guide therapeutic relationships, be restorative and so enable practitioners to deepen 'being' with patients and themselves. The potential benefits of engaging in supervision are briefly summarized in Box 6.4.

Box 6.4 Clinical supervision: the potential benefits

- Support practitioners whose work is often challenging and demanding (White et al 1998)
- Provide time for 'reflection on' practice aimed at improving patient care (Butterworth & Faugier 1992)
- Collegiate sharing of up-to-date practice (Bishop 1994)
- Clarify personal and professional issues and boundaries (Westland 1995)
- Clinical risk management tool (Tingle 1995)
- Guidance and support in fulfilling professional potential (Jones 1995)
- Acknowledge and celebrate 'potency' in therapeutic work (Mackereth 1997)
- Fine-tune the 'internal supervisor' by supporting reflection in practice (Jennings 1999)
- Experiential contribution to learning about supervisory roles and skills (Cutcliffe & Proctor 1998).

REFERENCES

Allitt Inquiry 1994 Independent inquiry chaired by Sir Cecil Clothier. HMSO, London

Bishop V 1994 Clinical supervision for an accountable profession. Nursing Times 90 (39): 35–37

Butterworth T Faugier J 1992 Clinical supervision and mentorship in nursing. Chapman and Hall, London

Butterworth T Bishop V Carson J 1996 First steps towards evaluating clinical supervision in nursing and health visiting – 1. Theory, policy and practice development. A review. Journal of Clinical Nursing 5: 127–132

Cromwell C Dryden S L Jones D Mackereth P A 1999 'Just the ticket': case studies, reflections and clinical supervision – part III. Complementary Therapies in Nursing & Midwifery 5 (2): 42–45

Cutcliffe J R Proctor B 1998 An alternative training approach to clinical supervision – Part 2. British Journal of Nursing 7 (6): 344–350

DoH 1993 Vision for the Future. National Management Executive, Department of Health, London

Faugier J Butterworth T 1994 Clinical supervision: a position paper, published by the School of Nursing Studies. University of Manchester, ISBN 1–898992–01–9

Hallberg I R Welander Hansson U Axelsson K 1994 Satisfaction with nursing care and work during a year of clinical supervision and individualized care. Comparison between two wards for the care of severely demented patients. Journal of Nursing Management 1: 297–307

Jennings S 1999 Theatre-based supervision: a supervision model for multidisciplinary supervisees. In: Tselikas-Portman E (ed) Supervision and dramatherapy. Jessica Kingsley, London

Johns C 1993 Professional supervision. Journal of Nursing Management 1: 9–18

Jones A 1995 Taking counsel. Nursing Times 91 (26): 28–29

Jones A 1996 Orem's self-care model and clinical supervision. International Journal of Palliative Nursing 2 (2): 77–83

Mackereth P A 1997 Clinical supervision for 'potent' practice. Complementary Therapies in Nursing and Midwifery 3: 38–41

Mackereth P A 1998 Body, relationship and sacred space. Complementary Therapies in Nursing and Midwifery 4 (5): 125–127

Mackereth P Gale E 1994 Touch/massage workshops – a pilot study. Complementary Therapies in Medicine 2: 93–98

McCallion H Baxter T 1995a Clinical supervision. How it works in the real world. Nursing Management 1 (9): 20–21

McCallion H Baxter T 1995b Clinical supervision, take it from the top. Nursing Management 2 (10): 9

McVey M L V-T 1996 Policy development. Complementary Therapies in Nursing and Midwifery 2: 41–46

Neil Cliffe Cancer Care Centre 1998 Protocols for the use of Complementary Therapies at the Neil Cliffe Cancer Care Centre. The Neil Cliffe Cancer Care Centre, Wythenshawe Hospital, Manchester

Penson J 1998 Complementary therapies: making a difference in palliative care. Complementary Therapies in Nursing and Midwifery 4 (3): 77–81

Pritchard T 1997 Supervision in practice. Nursing in Critical Care 2 (1): 34–37

Rankin-Box D 1997 Therapies in practice: a survey assessing nurses' use of complementary therapies. Complementary Therapies in Nursing and Midwifery 3: 92–99

Rodriguez R Goorapah D 1998 Clinical supervision for nurse teachers: the pertinent issues. British Journal of Nursing 7 (11): 663–669

Tingle J 1995 Clinical supervision is an effective risk management tool. British Journal of Nursing 4 (14): 794–795

UKCC 1992 The Scope of Professional Practice. UKCC, London.

UKCC 1995 Position Statement on Clinical Supervision for Nursing and Health Visiting. UKCC, London

Vickers A 1996 Massage and aromatherapy: a guide for health professionals. Chapman and Hall, London

Westland G 1995 An evolving model of supervision for biodynamic massage. Association of Holistic Biodynamic Massage Therapist Newsletter No. 4

White E Butterworth T Bishop V Carson J Jeacock J Clements A 1998 Clinical supervision: insider reports of a private world. Journal of Advanced Nursing 28 (1): 185–192

Yegdich T 1998 How not to do clinical supervision in nursing. Journal of Advanced Nursing 28 (1): 193–202

6 Research issues

Caroline Stevensen

INTRODUCTION

Many nurses who practise complementary therapies have not trained in research methodology. To these nurses, the thought of having to evaluate their complementary therapy practice in this way can be overwhelming. However, performing research in complementary therapies need not be as daunting as it first appears.

To justify the use of complementary therapies in nursing, as with complementary therapies in medicine and other areas of health care, an evidence base has become the watchword of the new millennium. In order to obtain this body of informed knowledge about the applicability and efficacy of complementary therapies in care, it is necessary to carry out appropriate research. There is ongoing discussion as to what forms this research may take and still ensure reliability. The place of the quantitative randomized controlled trial may be limited or inappropriate for answering questions raised by complementary therapy nursing research. Other qualitative methods may be more appropriate. As in any form of research the research question should determine the methodology not the other way round. The lack of competent research published about specific complementary therapies within nursing has meant that, in certain health care environments, these therapies are not currently practised. The role of research for the ongoing practice of complementary therapies within nursing is therefore crucial. This chapter will discuss a range of issues relating to the performance of research within complementary therapies in nursing care.

DEFINING RESEARCH

Research is simply finding out the answer to a question for which we do not already have an answer, for example:

1. Does aromatherapy reduce insomnia amongst elderly care patients?
2. Does the use of individualized relaxing music reduce analgesic needs in the post-surgical patient?
3. What is the effect of shiatsu on anxiety for post-cardiac surgery patients?

4. How do patients' perceptions of nursing care vary when a range of complementary therapies are available on the ward?

5. How do nurses view the introduction of massage onto the intensive care ward?

6. Why do nurses undertake training in reflexology?

It should be possible to ask only one question and to state it in a single phrase; the questions should immediately suggest the research design (Vickers 1995b).

Possible research design:

- Quantitative research: randomized controlled trials (RCT)
- Qualitative research
- Systematic review
- Audit
- Laboratory studies.

Quantitative research

In quantitative studies, questions of measurement are most easily undertaken questions (see question 1–3 mentioned above).

Ernst (1997) suggests that complementary therapies are perceived as effective or they would not be used in clinical practice. He goes on to say that the scientifically relevant question is whether complementary therapies are superior to placebo or sham interventions that have no specific effect. To answer this question the researcher must use a quantitative approach or RCT. However, it must be noted that there is a shift moving away from the idea that RCT is the only valid means of evaluating complementary therapies, despite existing pressure from orthodox medicine.

Qualitative research

Qualitative research focuses upon questions of meaning, motivation or social significance. Qualitative research design may be more appropriate for questions 4–6 mentioned above. Here, the format may be more of the structured interview with open-ended questions. Answers from research subjects may then be placed in different categories allowing for themes to emerge.

Systematic review

Other forms of research may be reviewing what research has been done before. This form of research may be called a systematic review or a meta-analysis of previously performed research trials.

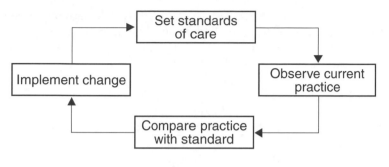

Figure 6.1 *An audit cycle.*

Audit

Audit in complementary therapies in nursing is the same process as audit in any other field of nursing. It takes an outcome snapshot of existing standards of care which can then be re-evaluated. The development of an audit cycle is a useful tool as standards of care can be set and the audit is a method of checking whether those standards are met (Fig. 6.1) (Vickers 1995a).

Laboratory studies

Laboratory studies consist of the largest proportion of medical research spending due to the large sums of money spent by the pharmaceutical industry. For nurses in clinical practice, these trials may not be appropriate. However, research nurses may find it possible to examine effects of complementary therapies in a laboratory setting, e.g. the effect of certain aromatic essential oils on levels of blood pressure and anxiety. Indeed, most research performed by scientists looking at the effects of essential oils for the pharmaceutical, cosmetic or food industries has been performed in this way.

BACKGROUND TO THE USE OF RESEARCH WITHIN COMPLEMENTARY THERAPIES IN NURSING

Ersser (1995) suggests those nurses using complementary therapies find it difficult to account adequately for their actions when information on safety and effectiveness is often inaccessible. Freshwater (1996) noted that complementary therapies in nursing were in danger of becoming disregarded due to lack of scientific research. This comment was based on a systematic review of the research literature on complementary therapies which concluded that much of the literature was either ignored or its merit questioned, for the simple reason that there was a lack of use of the RCT. Chabot's (1990) paper on the evaluation of holistic medicine identifies the difficulties in determining efficacy due to the variety of methods which were used to compare different types of therapy and the lack of familiarization with the model of holistic medicine.

Nurses have been brave enough to move away from the RCT to more qualitative methods which emphasize a greater degree of individuality, humanism, participation and interaction (Biley & Freshwater 2000). Indeed, nurses have begun to acknowledge the immense breadth and depth of nursing knowledge and practice and the need for different methods of measurement.

THE VALUE OF RESEARCH WITHIN NURSING

Whatever the background, both research and complementary therapies are now firmly part of nursing practice. This is a marriage that may rest uncomfortably with the nurse using complementary therapies who does not want to spend her already limited time on performing long and complex research trials when she could be spending that time with patients in the clinical setting. However, as we enter the next millennium, one thing is certain – the need for a sound evidence base will increase as the demand on health care resources becomes more competitive. Nurses will be required, at every turn, to have a good evidence base to justify the practice of complementary therapies. Rayner (1998) states that acupuncture only makes sense now that we understand endorphines, but that reflexology is not yet valid because we do not yet comprehend the mechanisms of its action. The development of this scientific basis, obtainable through research, will make sense of what is currently without explanation.

Audit is such a universally accepted practice in nursing that it should be relatively simple for most nurses to get some quality information about the standards of care being currently offered by complementary therapies within their setting.

KEY ISSUES IN COMPLEMENTARY THERAPY RESEARCH TRIAL

Steps to take:

- What is the research question?
- Is it relevant?
- Is it a feasible study?
- What literature is available regarding previous research in that field? (The reading of journal abstracts can be misleading as they

rarely provide sufficient information to decide whether or not the research was properly conducted. Claims made by authors may not be substantiated in the body of the paper.)

- Critically appraise the previous research performed: sample size, appropriateness of control groups, randomization, are the groups comparable at baseline, blinding, appropriate outcome measures, are all patients accounted for at the end of the trial, appropriate statistics used, generalizable results to other groups or settings (Vickers 1995b).

- What research design or methodology lends itself to investigate the question?

- Is collaboration possible?

- Writing the research proposal.

- Is there funding available?

- Is ethical committee approval required?

- Have ethical considerations of the patients been observed (e.g. understanding of the research, informed written consent, right to privacy, maintenance of dignity, confidentiality, freedom from harm, anonymity, self-determination)?

- Has consent been sought from relevant parties?

- Have relevant staff and personnel been informed about the project?

- Has a pilot study been performed to test the validity of the measurement tools?

- Collecting the data.

- Analysis of the results – are the methods chosen valid and reliable?

- Writing up – who is your target audience? (Include a summary of the research and its major findings, an introduction of the subject and literature review, methods including sample selection, study design, outcome measures, results, discussion including limitation of the study, how the research contributes to the wider body of knowledge in the field, further research that could be performed.)

- Publication: for research to be of value, the results must be published in a relevant journal. Journals such as *Complementary Therapies in Nursing and Midwifery* or *Complementary Therapies in Medicine* may be appropriate.

PRACTICAL CONSIDERATIONS

Knowledge, skills, supervision, time and money seem to be the basic considerations required for the performance of any research, and the field of complementary therapies within nursing is not excluded from this. It is important to note that enthusiasm alone does not perform research and to obtain sound training in research skills is paramount before any nurse commences such an endeavour. It is also most important to have a supervisor in the form of an experienced researcher in that field to guide the research process and prevent valuable time and energy being wasted. It is not advisable to embark on research without adequate time or sufficient provision of funds. There are various grant-giving bodies which may be able to offer some financial support for research. This is why a well-prepared research proposal is necessary to compete for these funds. The quickest way not to complete a research project is to be 'up against it' both with time and money. Get advice from a number of different experienced complementary therapy researchers before a lot of time and effort is committed to the project.

Summary

Recent developments in complementary nursing research are both exciting and innovative. Nurses now have the knowledge and the courage to break away from traditional research designs that may not fit the broad humanistic aspects of complementary therapy nursing research. Depending on the research question, a variety of designs may be chosen, from the quantitative method of RCT to more innovative forms of qualitative research.

The climate is ripe for a rapid growth of quality complementary nursing research; without this, the permission for nurses to practise a range of complementary therapies in their clinical setting may not be granted as the movement towards evidence-based medicine beds down into current health culture. Let us hope that we do not limit the pioneering and visionary aspects to our complementary therapy nursing whilst we are allowing this process to take place.

REFERENCES

Biley F, Freshwater D 2000 Trends in nursing and midwifery research and the need for change in complementary therapy research. Complementary Therapies in Nursing and Midwifery (in press)

Chabot P 1990 The evaluation of holistic care. International Revue of Community Development (Revue-International-d' action-communautaire) 24 (64): 109–114

Ernst E 1997 Evidence-based complementary medicine. Complementary Therapies in Nursing and Midwifery 3 (2): 42–45

Ersser S 1995 Complementary therapies and nursing research: issues and practicalities. Complementary Therapies in Nursing and Midwifery 1 (2): 44–50

Freshwater D 1996 Complementary therapies and research in nursing practice. Nursing Standard 10 (38): 43–45

Rayner C 1998 Medicine: magic or myth? Complementary Therapies in Nursing and Midwifery 4 (2): 33–34

Vickers A 1995a A basic introduction to medical research – Part 2: An overview of different research methods. Complementary Therapies in Nursing and Midwifery. 1 (4): 113–117

Vickers A 1995b A basic introduction to medical research – Part 3: What can the practitioner do? Complementary Therapies in Nursing and Midwifery 1 (5): 143–147

FURTHER READING – JOURNALS

Fisher P 1995 The development of research methodology in homoeopathy. Complementary Therapies in Nursing and Midwifery 1 (6): 168–174

Fitter M J, Thomas K J 1997 Evaluating complementary therapies for use in the national health service: 'Horses for Courses' – Part 1: The design challenge. Complementary Therapies in Medicine 5 (2): 90–93

Furham A F 1994 The Barum effect in medicine. Complementary Therapies in Medicine 2 (1): 1–4

Thomas K J Fitter M J 1997 Evaluating complementary therapies for use in the national health service: 'Horses for Courses' – Part 2: Alternative research strategies. Complementary Therapies in Medicine 5 (2): 94–98

Vickers A 1995 A basic introduction to medical research – Part 1: What is research and why do it? Complementary Therapies in Nursing and Midwifery. 1 (3): 67–96

Vickers A and Rees R 1995 Literature searching in complementary medical research. Complementary Therapies in Nursing and Midwifery 1 (6): 175–177

USEFUL ADDRESSES

The British Library Science Reference and Information Service (SRIS)
9 Kean Street
London WC2

The British Library Reading Room
Great Russell Street London WC1
Tel: 020 7323 7676
Reader's ticket required

Royal College of Nursing Library
20 Cavendish Square
London W1M 0AB
Tel: 020 7409 3333
Open to members only

Homoeopathic Information Service
Glasgow Homoeopathic Hospital
1000 Great Western Road
Glasgow G21 0NR
Tel: 0141 337 1824

British Medical Library Information Service
Boston Spa
Wetherby
West Yorkshire LS23 7BQ
Tel: 01937 546 039
Can supply photocopies of most papers at a charge of £4.50 per paper

7 Ethical and legal issues

Julie Stone

INTRODUCTION

Enthusiasm for complementary therapies amongst nurses has never been higher. Taking the opportunity to re-introduce elements of holistic care into work which has become ever more technological, nurses are introducing a range of therapies into their practice. As the evidence base for complementary medicine grows, and more and more patients are requesting complementary therapies from their orthodox health professionals, there is increasing interest in, and support for, integration with the NHS. However, concerns about lack of regulation, variations in standards of training and practice and a paucity of efficacy data are hampering moves towards wholesale introduction of these therapies. Indeed, there is something of a backlash against the introduction of complementary therapies in an unsafe, unregulated fashion. It is critical, therefore, that nurses work within legal and ethical boundaries. This chapter will look at some of the main ethical and legal issues raised by nurses introducing complementary therapies into their practice.

LEGAL AND ETHICAL ISSUES RAISED BY NURSES USING CAM THERAPIES

Appropriate training

It should go without saying that nurses should not introduce complementary therapies into their work unless they have been adequately trained. As therapies professionalize, growing numbers of courses are being externally validated through universities, and nurses should satisfy themselves that the course is of an appropriate length and depth, with both theoretical and practical aspects of training. Nurses need to make sure that they have satisfactorily completed a training course recognized by a credible professional body and that their training will allow them to become registered with a credible professional body.

Ensuring competent practice

Competent practice should ensure that patients are not harmed through the use of complementary therapies. The notion of competence has ethical and legal implications. Incompetent practice is unethical, as it means that the patient will not derive benefit (*beneficence*) from the treatment and may indeed be harmed (*non-maleficence*). A patient who is harmed may sue the nurse or the hospital. At a time when the NHS is spending millions on settlements in legal actions, risk management has become a major concern. NHS managers may be very wary of allowing nurses to introduce complementary therapies unless they are confident that nurses are working within protocols, to an appropriately high standard and carry professional indemnity insurance.

Defining what constitutes competent practice within complementary medicine is extremely controversial. Unlike statutory health professions, where practice standards are determined through nationally imposed core curricula under the aegis of a statutory education committee, many complementary therapies have yet to define common educational standards and core competencies. Therapies commonly used by nurses, including aromatherapy, reflexology, therapeutic touch and massage therapy, are not statutorily regulated in the UK at present, meaning that anyone can set themselves up in practice and call themselves a therapist with little or no training and standards of training and practice within these therapies vary significantly.

Whilst several therapies in the UK have been working towards producing National Occupational Standards (including aromatherapy, hypnotherapy, homeopathy and reflexology), the fragmentation and diversity within many other therapies is so great that it is almost impossible to define what competence amounts to in any particular therapy, beyond agreeing on the barest minimum standards.

Working within limits of competence

As registered health professionals, nurses in the UK are bound to work within the standards set down by the United Kingdom Central Council for Nursing, Midwifery and Health Visiting (UKCC). The Council's *Guidelines on Professional Practice* recognize the growing popularity of CAM therapies, but state:

> *'It is vitally important that you ensure that the introduction of any of these therapies to your practice is always in the best interests and safety of the patients and clients.'*   (UKCC 1996)

The guidance continues that registered nurses must be convinced of the relevance of using the therapy and must be able to justify it in the particular circumstance.

Using complementary therapies has consequences for the overall management of a patient, particularly in the event of a mishap, so nurses should discuss the use of complementary therapies with medical and other members of the health care team caring for the particular patient. Although most of the complementary interventions nurses use in a hospital setting are supplementary to the orthodox care patients are receiving, nurses who view their interventions as genuinely alternative to the conventional approach may find themselves philosophically at odds with the treatment regimen which has been prescribed for the patient by their doctors. The BMA, in its book *Complementary Medicine. New Approaches to Good Practice* (BMA 1993) states:

> '...it is essential that non-conventional therapists should not alter the medication or treatment prescribed for patients by their medical practitioner.'

Quality assurance as an ethical and legal issue

The concept of clinical governance puts quality assurance at the heart of health care. The creation in the UK of the National Institute of Clinical Excellence and the Commission for Health Improvement demonstrates a commitment to the principle that all health interventions should benefit patients and be cost-effective. In the past, quality concerns have been an obstacle to NHS employers interested in providing complementary therapies. Hospital/Trust employers should always ensure that staff offering CAM therapies are appropriately qualified to do so, and should require nurses to have the following:

- Proof of qualifications (the therapist's certificate; a copy of the syllabus studied; examination results; evidence of continuing professional development)
- Sufficient professional indemnity insurance
- Evidence of registration with an appropriate professional body which produces a Code of Ethics, requires members to carry insurance and has a disciplinary mechanism.

WORKING WITHIN SCOPE OF EMPLOYMENT

Unless specifically negotiated, the use of complementary therapies is unlikely to fall within the nurse's usual scope of employment. This places the nurse in a potentially vulnerable position, in terms of employment, professional and legal responsibilities. Nurses intending to incorporate therapeutic interventions should only do so with the support, and in the full knowledge of, their line manager, preferably in accordance with an established and agreed protocol. Failure to do so could result in the nurse being subject to disciplinary action by employers. It could also possibly result in misconduct procedures brought by the UKCC, who state in their guidance:

'If a complaint is made against you, we can call you to account for any activities carried out outside conventional practice. You should carefully consider the content and status of any courses which you undertake and how you promote yourself.' (UKCC 1996)

In other words, whilst the UKCC do not actively discourage nurses from using complementary therapies as part of their work, personal accountability is of the utmost concern, and the onus on ensuring safety is placed firmly on practitioners.

LACK OF EVIDENCE BASE

As nurses using complementary therapies are trying to bring about some benefit to patients, be it psychological or physical, how can they be sure, in the absence of an evidence base for most therapies, that their efforts are worthwhile and that the complementary therapies that they are offering are causing net benefit? All nurses, as part of their professional responsibilities, should be committed to evidence-based practice, yet there is a dearth of reliable, published research within complementary medicine. As health professionals trained in research methodology and inculcated in scientific medicine, nurses have a critical function in auditing their use of complementary therapies and, wherever possible, adding to the research literature.

PROBLEMS GAINING CONSENT

As a matter of law and ethics, nurses must obtain a patient's consent to any intervention. This serves to protect the patient's autonomy and to protect the nurse from an allegation of battery for unauthorized touching. It has been argued that if the evidence is not there, how can nurses really tell a patient what the risks are going to be (Ernst 1996)? Nurses must also remember that, whereas doctors only tend to think of informing patients about physical risks of treatment, patients need to know that complementary therapies may affect them on a physical, emotional or even spiritual level.

POSSIBLE SCOPE TO CAUSE HARM

Although there are relatively few reported incidents of serious harm, nurses should not assume that complementary therapies, however 'natural' or non-invasive, are universally safe. In unskilled hands, all therapeutic interventions have the capacity to cause harm, and the RCN have expressed particular concerns about the dangers of inappropriate use of aromatherapy oils. The ethical duty to avoid harm involves ensuring that any product or equipment used is safe and well-maintained, and also requires that nurses themselves are in good physical and psychological health.

WHETHER HOSPITAL/NHS TRUST WOULD INDEMNIFY IN EVENT OF MISHAP

So far, there has been almost no litigation arising out of the use of complementary medicine either in the UK or in the USA; this is remarkable given its wide usage. This seems to be due to the trusting relationship that patients develop with complementary practitioners over a period of time and the empathy which evolves out of a holistic, one-to-one relationship. A concern is that many of the current barriers to suing a complementary practitioner in a private patient setting would disappear if the patient suffered harm as part of their treatment given by a nurse in the NHS. Rather than feeling reluctant to sue a known individual, a patient who did suffer harm might feel more inclined to instigate litigation or a complaint against a faceless NHS Hospital/Trust's legal department.

Where would this leave the nurse? Ordinarily, the Hospital/Trust would be vicariously liable for the acts or omissions of members of their staff (Stone & Matthews 1996). However, if we consider the case of a nurse who caused harm to a patient by using an undiluted aromatherapy oil directly to the skin, or massaging a patient at risk of deep vein thrombosis, it would be unlikely that her employing Hospital/Trust would be prepared to indemnify the nurse, as it would say that such action was acting outside the scope of employment. As such, the nurse would be held personally accountable, and it would be unwise for any nurse to start providing CAM therapies without informing her line manager of her intention and obtaining appropriate professional indemnity insurance.

WHY SUING MAY NOT BE AN APPROPRIATE COURSE OF ACTION

In legal terms, a nurse owes a patient a duty to act with reasonable skill. If this duty is breached and the patient suffers harm, an action in negligence may arise. The level of duty owed is called the *standard of care*. The problem is that in the absence of any existing case law, it is very difficult to determine exactly the standard of care owed by a nurse. In the absence of nationally agreed standards, it is impossible to predict with any degree of certainty what level of duty of care a court would impose upon a nurse practising a complementary therapy in the event of a mishap. The standard of care is that of the 'ordinarily competent practitioner', which means, in effect, that nurses should work within the guidelines set down by the relevant therapy's professional body.

If a nurse does harm a patient through use of complementary therapies, the law is unlikely to provide satisfactory redress. Law is poor at responding to harm that is not of a serious, lasting, physical nature. Hopefully, it would be rare for any nurse to inflict that degree of harm. This may leave the patient without a remedy for harm which is of a less serious, more transient nature, but which nonetheless causes the patient to suffer. Similarly, it would be highly unlikely that a patient could seek a legal remedy against a nurse who caused considerable emotional distress by over-enthusiastic use of counselling techniques, for example, as the law is slow to compensate for harms that it cannot see or measure. A patient or their family, could, however, bring a formal complaint against the nurse through the NHS complaints system, which may lead to employers questioning the further provision of such techniques.

Summary

Complementary therapies can benefit patients but they can also cause harm. Whatever the regulatory status of the therapies they are using, nurses must ensure they are working within ethical and legal boundaries. Nurses are fully accountable for their professional practice and must ensure that their acts or omissions do not cause patients harm. By working ethically and legally, nurses should be able to provide a safe framework in which patients can receive, and nurses can deliver, therapies that will hopefully

REFERENCES

BMA 1993 Complementary medicine. New approaches to good practice. British Medical Association/Oxford University Press, Oxford

Ernst E 1996 The ethics of complementary medicine. Journal of Medical Ethics 22: 197–198

Stone J and Matthews J 1996 Complementary medicine and the law. Oxford University Press, Oxford

UKCC, 1996 Guidelines for Professional Practice. United Kingdom Central Council for Nursing, Midwifery and Health Visiting, London

FURTHER READING

Cohen M 1998 Complementary and alternative medicine: legal boundaries and regulatory perspectives. Johns Hopkins University Press, New York

Dimond B 1998 The legal aspects of complementary therapy practice. Churchill Livingstone, Edinburgh

Stone J and Matthews J 1996 Complementary medicine and the law. Oxford University Press, Oxford

8 Integrated health care: implications for nursing practice

Angela Avis

INTRODUCTION

This chapter will explore professional and practical issues involved with the integration of complementary therapies into patient care in general and nursing in particular. A trawl through dictionaries suggests that to integrate is to combine a part(s) into a whole. At first glance this says nothing about the relationship of the various parts within the whole. The key concept in relation to the integration of complementary therapies that most dictionaries go on to describe is that the parts come into equal membership of a 'whole'. Integration in these terms is not just about the whimsical addition of parts (complementary therapies), it is about a systematic process that reviews the 'whole' (nursing care), and adjusts its constituent parts in line with therapeutic objectives. Any additional parts are integrated because equal value is ascribed to them in relation to fulfilling the objectives of the 'whole'. This means, however, that the relative size of the contribution of any of the parts of the whole will have to be adjusted because the 'whole' has a definitive boundary. Equal value does not mean equal size of the parts.

Complementary therapies will need to be shown to be cost-effective if they are to be part of the NHS provision. The therapeutic potential of any complementary therapy will be measured by the same criteria as the orthodox provision. In relation to the integration of complementary therapies within nursing, this will mean that other aspects of care will be affected. Therefore the use of a therapy will have to be justified as an alternative therapeutic option, using appropriate criteria. If a therapy were to be used in a complementary but additional way, then there would need to be an increase in resources.

INTEGRATED HEALTH CARE

Integrated health care describes the development of high quality health services that effectively integrate the best of orthodox and complementary health care and has grown from the work of the Foundation for Integrated Medicine (FIM). This organization has been formed from working groups set up at the suggestion of the Prince of Wales, to consider the current positions of orthodox, complementary and alternative medicine in the UK and how appropriate and possible it would be for them to work more closely together (FIM 1997). Integrated approaches reflect different models of care, spanning primary and secondary sectors. The approach is not simply concerned with techniques. Attention is given to the beliefs and values under-pinning health care. So, for example, integrated health care would mean adopting a holistic approach to patient care by giving adequate attention to the psychological, social, environmental and spiritual aspects of health care delivery. In addition the patient-centred nature of health care would be enhanced by valuing and developing collabo-rative relationships among staff from a wide range of professions. The integrated health care approach reflects a desire for radical thinking in the restructuring and development of services that incorporate these values and combine new therapeutic options. The intention is to reform health services in such a way that they offer the prospect of meeting health needs that have otherwise been poorly met by the existing services (FIM 1997). The aim is not only to increase the thera-peutic repertoire in order to aid recovery and rehabilitation but also to provide those in need with additional support when coping with chronic illness or impending death.

Integrated health care may be delivered through many different models of health care provision. The following list gives some examples but is not exhaustive:

- A complementary therapist may be contracted to provide a specific service

- Complementary therapists may offer a service on a voluntary basis

- Orthodox practitioners may directly refer patients to an independent complementary therapist

- A GP practice may offer sessions from a range of therapists who are funded as part of the practice team

- Orthodox health professionals, having undertaken training, may offer certain techniques or treatments from a therapy as an integral part of their practice

- Some orthodox practitioners may be able to offer a therapy in its entirety as a separate service, within their NHS contracted hours

- Carers who have skills in complementary therapies could be encouraged to use them with the people they care for and they may teach health professionals simple techniques so that continuity is maintained.

These are only a few examples of delivery models and they demonstrate imagination and the need for discussion and collaboration with medical and other members of the health care team (UKCC 1996). It is apparent that there is scope for the development of many different delivery models in response to the unique aspects of any given community or clinical environment.

Important practice, education, ethico-legal and research issues arise from the push to integrate complementary therapies into clinical nursing practice. The incentive for improving or enhancing nursing practice in relation to the use of complementary therapies must start with valuing nursing as a therapeutic activity, and progress into finding ways to generate policies and protocols to guide and support nurses in the safe and effective use of complementary therapies within their everyday work. In embracing complementary therapies, nurses need to consider keeping any activity focused on the phenomenon of the therapeutic relationship that is at the heart of nursing. Without this emphasis there is a danger that the therapies will become 'quick-fix' acts in themselves, devoid of therapeutic meaning. This will lead to complementary therapies becoming little more than new tasks to be used clinically in certain generic cases, without recognizing and respecting the uniqueness of either the patient or the therapy (Bay 1995). Integration is about giving equal value to the various parts of the therapeutic nursing repertoire.

COMPLEMENTARY THERAPIES IN NURSING

When exploring the background to the integration of complementary therapies into nursing a number of questions arise. For example, are nurses trying to integrate the entire range of complementary therapies within nursing practice or simply a few selected therapies? It would be difficult to integrate all therapies into nursing practice. First, the use of a complementary therapy should be based on sound and substantial evidence of the expected therapeutic outcome if nurses are not to be accused of following the latest fad or fashion (Rayner 1998, Hehir 1999). This would reduce the range considerably (Vickers 1996, Ernst 1997). Another restricting factor would be in selecting therapies that could be appropriately included in what is currently defined as the scope of nursing practice. For instance, osteopathy and chiropractic are highly specialized and specific therapies that focus on the body structure using touch and manipulation. They are 'complete systems' (Pietroni 1990) in that they include diagnosis and treatment. A recent informal survey undertaken by the Royal College of Nursing (Rankin-Box 1997) has indicated that massage, aromatherapy and reflexology are the therapies most widely used within nursing. These therapies are described as having a 'therapeutic modality' in the classification of complementary therapies outlined by Pietroni, which would suggest that they are therapies that would enhance nursing care. Another concern is whether the focus is upon integration of a 'total' therapy or of a particular technique that is part of a therapy. Is this integration or 'fragmentation'? Will the use of a complementary therapy technique become integrated as a seamless part of nursing or just another fragmented task that is abandoned when workloads increase? These questions are a necessary part of the debate around the scope of professional practice that must take place prior to substantive integration.

For many nurses the practice of complementary therapies seems very attractive. This may be due to an awareness of the focused time complementary therapists spend with their clients, in contrast to the hustle and bustle of the clinical environment. Many nurses feel that they could do so much more for their patients if they only had more time. This can lead to a tendency to equate the use of a complementary therapy within practice as a device to magically expand time and therefore the quality of the care given. However, if a complementary therapy or technique is to be used within the clinical environment then something else will probably not be done. Newbeck (1986) suggested that trying to integrate complementary therapies into nursing practice without fundamental changes in other aspects, such as valuing the nurse–patient relationship, would be like trying to ice an uncooked cake. Complementary therapies should not be used as a substitute for good basic nursing care. There is an argument to be made that the effective and appropriate integration of complementary therapies within nursing is about practice that is complex and sophisticated. It requires skills in critical reflection, decision-making, the management of change and in-depth knowledge of the clinical area. In addition the nurse must undertake training in the particular therapy that is of sufficient rigour, with a substantial period of consolidation, to ensure safe and effective clinical care. The implication could be that nurses should not be considering using complementary therapies until they have consolidated their practice as a nurse.

The decision to use a complementary therapy may be valid but it should be made using a systematic process, exploring different therapeutic options within the nursing repertoire that are always in the best interests and safety of patients and clients (UKCC 1996).

GENERALIST OR SPECIALIST?

Continuity of care is an important issue and is of particular significance in relation to the use of complementary therapies within nursing. In the past perhaps only one nurse in any particular clinical area initiated the use of complementary therapies. Motivation has been complex, sometimes bordering on the evangelical. The nurse may not have been in a position of authority, or aware of organizational or political constraints, and therefore was unable to influence the culture of their clinical area. Without effective management of change, complementary therapies have tended to be offered in a piecemeal way. The availability of limited nursing staff trained in therapies restricts patient access to complementary therapies and impedes the development of an equitable service.

EDUCATION AND TRAINING

Education is a key factor in relation to safe and effective nursing care and raises many issues, in particular the uncertainty about the relationship between professional nursing practice and existing sources of education and expertise in complementary therapies. There should be debate about the appropriate education required in any particular therapy when integrated into a clinical setting, with careful consideration given to the content and status of any particular course (UKCC 1996). There is a need to link levels of competency to clinical practice and to be explicit about the scope of practice (UKCC 1996). Questions are then raised with regard to the educational standards of the numerous professional bodies that currently exist within the complementary therapy field and whether as nurses it is appropriate to draw a distinction between education needed for independent practice and that needed for the use of complementary therapies in the care of sick people. It is important to recognize professional responsibilities involving the individual nurse being held accountable for their actions. By acknowledging the wide range of health needs and delivery models by which services can be offered, there is a recognition of the different educational needs of practitioners.

Summary

A qualified nurse must work within the framework of the UKCC Code of Professional Conduct, and this is as true for the use of complementary therapies as for any other form of nursing care. If there is to be true integration the delivery process must include the following aspects:

- Nurses must undertake substantial training in any therapy, including a period of consolidation, if they are intending to deliver the therapy themselves
- Nurses must be specific about the therapeutic outcomes they are seeking to achieve, developing an articulate rationale
- A structure for competent and consistent supervision and mentorship should be available

Summary Cont'd

- Awareness of current research should be demonstrated and nurses encouraged to increase the evidence base using a range of research methodologies
- Appropriate tools should be developed in order to audit the outcome and quality of care
- Planning should be undertaken collaboratively with other members of the health care team
- When external therapists are involved there must be agreed protocols that enable the nurse to be accountable for the standard of care given by that therapist
- Policies and protocols must be developed that provide safe and effective care that integrates the use of complementary therapies. These will include issues such as informed consent and risk management.

This may seem like a daunting list but if equal value is to be placed on the therapeutic potential of complementary therapies within nursing, there are no short cuts. Considerable commitment is involved. In this way the use of complementary therapies within nursing will result in true integration that uses the best of orthodox and complementary approaches to provide high quality nursing care that is appropriate, safe and effective.

REFERENCES

Bay F 1995 Complementary therapies – just another task? Complementary Therapies in Nursing and Midwifery 1 (1): 34–36

Ernst E 1997 Evidenced-based complementary medicine. Complementary Therapies in Nursing and Midwifery 3 (1): 42–45

FIM 1997 Integrated healthcare – a way forward for the next five years? Foundation for Integrated Medicine, London

Hehir B 1999 Opiate of the people. Nursing Times 95 (32): 30–31

Newbeck I 1986 How holistic therapies can be used in nursing. Second Holistic Nursing Conference, City University, London

Pietroni P 1990 The greening of medicine. Victor Gollancz, London

Rankin-Box D 1997 Therapies in practice: a survey assessing nurses' use of complementary therapies. Complementary Therapies in Nursing and Midwifery 3 (2): 92–99

Rayner C 1998 Medicine: magic or myth? Complementary Therapies in Nursing and Midwifery 4 (1): 33–34

UKCC 1996 Guidelines for Professional Practice. United Kingdom Central Council for Nursing, Midwifery and Health Visiting, London

Vickers A 1996 Criticism, scepticism and complementary medicine. In: Vickers A (ed) Examining complementary medicine. Stanley Thornes, Cheltenham.

9 Complementary therapies and nursing models

Fiona Mantle

INTRODUCTION

With the advent of integrated nursing, i.e. the integration of complementary therapies into nursing care, it is time to ask whether existing nursing models adequately address this nursing development. This chapter explores a number of definitions of nursing as offered by prominent nurse theorists from which their models have evolved, and establishes their congruence with some of the philosophies inherent in the majority of complementary therapies. The approach undertaken by the models will be analysed, specifically addressing the concept of holism. Finally, a new approach to holistic care will be offered based upon the work of Benner (1984) and personal construct theory (Kelly 1955).

Micozzi (1996) suggested that the key attributes of complementary therapies include the concepts of vitalism, or vital force, in the promotion of self-healing, with an emphasis on wellness and the empowerment of the client. Other factors include the concept of taking responsibility for one's own health, the partnership between therapist and client and the encouragement of self-help, which might include adjustment of the environment and the revision of lifestyle. In their reviews of complementary therapies, Trevelyan & Booth (1994), Fulder (1996) and Micozzi (1996) discuss a number of therapies which enshrine these principles and in which treatment is based on re-establishing equilibrium through the re-balancing of the body's vital energy to promote self-healing.

At this point a comparison of the principal factors espoused in nursing definitions and models of similarities between complementary therapies and nursing is worth considering. For example, Florence Nightingale noted that each human individual has vital, recuperative powers to deal with disease and that the goal of nursing is to place the individual in the best possible condition for nature to act upon them. Similarly, Henderson's (1966) definition states:

'That the unique function of the nurse was to assist the individual, sick or well in the performance of those activities contributing to health or its recovery (or to a peaceful death) that he [sic] would perform unaided if he had the necessary strength, will or knowledge and to do this in such a way as to help him gain independence as rapidly as possible.'

In line with Nightingale, there is an emphasis upon the facilitation of independence and health promotion.

In 1984, Roy took a systems approach suggesting each body system was in continuous interaction with the environment and aiming to maintain a level of homeostasis. She claimed that the function of the nurse is the promotion of adaptive responses in the client by manipulating the stimuli impinging on the person so that adaptive responses are promoted. This could be achieved by teaching the patient how to adjust to changing stimuli in order to achieve equilibrium and engender the promotion of self-healing leading to a higher level of wellness.

Orem's (1985) self-care concept explicitly states the premise that adults have the innate impetus to care for themselves and thus initiate activities that promote self-care, health and well-being. In common with other models of nursing she emphasized the role of the nurse as facilitator and change agent. She further suggested that nursing is not a tangible commodity but is dependent on situations as they present themselves. None of the goals of nursing, as defined by these theorists, could be achieved without the nurse working in partnership with the patient or the patient's active contribution to the goal.

All nursing models address these concepts, some more explicitly than others. In all models nurses are depicted as facilitators or agents of change working with the client towards a level of wellness. It can be seen from this that nursing and complementary therapies, to a greater or lesser extent, share a number of common approaches.

Central to the integration of complementary therapies into nursing care and the use of nursing models is the concept of holism. It could be argued that all nursing models propose a holistic approach. Sharma (1994) suggested that holism may come in a variety of degrees and divided the concept into weak and strong forms. The weakest form involves identifying the patient's symptoms as part of a total health profile encompassing mind, body and spirit. The stronger form takes this concept a stage further and includes the previously discussed aspects such as empowering the patient by encouragement and education to take on more responsibility for their own health. Boschma (1994) echoes this by stressing that holism includes a major emphasis on self-help and self-awareness with the person accepting responsibility for their own health and well-being. Holism involves the promotion of healthier habits to increase wellness and the idea that illness is seen as a potential for growth and the gaining of self-knowledge. Of particular importance is the development of the therapeutic relationship between client and practitioner to facilitate healing. Watson (1979) saw the nurse as a catalyst assisting clients to grow and change, and Neuman (1982), speaking in the context of nursing, suggested that this relationship is a partnership within which both the client and practitioner can grow and develop. Ham-Ying's (1993) more recent analysis of the term 'holism' in the context of nursing found that it had two common usages: a personal view, i.e. the person seen as a holistic being, and holism as an approach to nursing care. She also highlighted a number of variations in definition, but argued that a key concept was the ideology that people are more than the sum of their parts and not a collection of sub-systems as defined by a bio/psycho/social being approach. However, other definitions of holism have advocated a different approach. Newbeck & Rowe (1986), in their essay on holism in nursing, wrote that '"holistic" nursing means offering an extended range of interventions to the clients ... such as: massage, relaxation therapy, meditation, reflexology and acupuncture'. This concept of holism has led Todd (1990) to maintain that many people now tend to define holism as a treatment modality, such as the complementary therapies, rather than a philosophy, but she suggests that true holism is 'the feelings and perspectives of holism, rather than the tools of practice, that define the approach.' She also claims, as do Vincent & Furnham (1997), that complementary therapies are not intrinsically holistic, although Buckle (1993) noted that modern discourse tends to intimate that 'holism is rapidly becoming a pseudonym ... for complementary'.

HOLISM IN PRACTICE

In 1971, Levine published the first article in which the term 'holistic nursing' was used. She described nursing thus:

> 'To many nurses the concept of holism is the central tenet in distinguishing nursing from medicine, since it emphasised the role of the nurse as one of viewing each patient as a complete and complex being in contrast to the reductionalist approach of medicine.'

Modern nurse theorists went on to emphasize this comprehensive approach to patients, defining the professional role as patient-orientated with a major emphasis on self-help and self-awareness. Early nursing theorists such as Rogers (1970) and Levine (1983) describe people in terms of their wholeness and as beings inseparable from their environments. Levine specifically noted that the fundamental concept of human life was holistic; in contrast, Roy's (1974) definition of holism presented a classic view of people as bio/psycho/social adaptive beings. Around the same time, Neuman (1974) used the terms physiologic, coniocultural, psychologic developmental beings.

Other perspectives include those of Orem (1985) who saw people as functioning biologically, symbolically and socially, while Roper et al (1985) echo Roy's bio/psyco/social definition. However, Korbet & Folan (1990) have suggested that these definitions, whilst attempting to be an encompassing view of the person, do in fact persist in defining human beings as an aggregation of their component sub-systems rather than a gestalt; the view that the person is more than the sum of their parts. Thus they unwittingly perpetuate the reductionalist view. The authors go on to suggest that nurses often believe that they are functioning under a holistic philosophy simply because the theory uses the word (Korbet & Folan 1990).

This is made manifest when translating nursing models into nursing practice using the nursing process which employs a mechanistic approach. Benner (1984) proposed that the reliance on nursing models was a feature of the novice and that, as experience is gained, nurses tend to move away from a prescribed approach to a more intellectually creative one. This is in contrast to Marks-Maran (1995) who suggested that in fact nursing seems to want conceptual models to be 'finished packages, perfect and complete', whereas in reality conceptual models, by their very nature, should be constantly evolving. What might be the answer here is an individual model of nursing unique to the nurse using it. Pearson & Vaughan (1986) suggest that 'nursing may be seen as a very large collection of concepts' that would be related to what people thought was important in nursing, although they admit that nurses may not be very good at expressing them. On a similar note, Kershaw (1992) discusses adopting a nursing model that is closely related to the nurse's self-image, one that she points out 'is unique and that this develops rather than inhibits the application of the nursing model'. Kershaw's is a particularly conducive solution since the nurse would feel more comfortable with this model rather than with one initiated by others.

So are nursing models suitable for use in integrated nursing care? The answer, based on Smut's definition of holism, is 'not entirely'. What is needed perhaps, is a model or system of nursing based on Benner (1984) and developed from Kershaw (1992) which directly addresses the therapeutic relationship by taking into account both the patient's and the nurse's concepts of nursing. This could be achieved by the adoption of 'personal construct theory' as a system of nursing. Thus, the model of care would be defined by both nurse and patient.

PERSONAL CONSTRUCT THEORY AS NURSING MODEL

Personal construct theory is based on the work of George Kelly (1955) who stated that we are all scientists: we form hypotheses about the world around us, test them out against reality and modify our constructs accordingly. They represent our personal view of life, will develop and change over our life's span as we gain experience and become an integral part of our self-concept. This is essentially a practical view of reality in that the concept of reality is individual and is constantly evolving over time. So, as situations change, the construct may be adapted or even discarded. It can be seen from this that reality can only be investigated by discovering how human beings perceive it. Because Kelly's theory is essentially focused on how people make sense of their private world, we are looking at its relevance and possible application to nursing. Kelly believed that since human beings are more than a montage of motivations, emotions and cognition (and we could add spirituality) his theory is an integrated gestalt and a truly holistic approach to understanding people. He stated:

> 'In talking about experience I have been careful not to use either of the terms, "emotion" or "affective". I have been equally careful not to invoke the notion of "cognition" … When one so divides the experience of man [sic] it becomes difficult to make the most of the holistic aspirations that may infuse the science of psychology with new life' (Kelly 1966, p 140).

Thus, Kelly refuted the reductionist approach, i.e. human beings as a group of sub-systems, instead taking a view of people which would have a high enough level of abstraction to embrace all human behaviour, combining the mind/body/spirit in the same psychological terms. It was a representation of self in its entirety.

Nurses coming into nursing have an individualistic view of the profession which is entirely their own and is interpreted through their constructs of nursing. For example, one nurse's view may be highly humanistic whilst another is more pragmatic.

These constructs undergo modification over time. Patients, too, have constructs of nursing which may not be made evident with existing models of care. It is the meeting and interaction of these constructs with the nurse's which may result in some adjustment of the respective constructs by both nurse and patient. From this it can be seen that each nurse has a unique model of nursing which is holistic (by Kelly's definition) as well as being dynamic and constantly evolving. The model develops during nurse training and continues to evolve during a professional lifetime as a part of self-development and awareness education and experience. Benner (1984) suggested that there is another body of nursing knowledge (other than static models) which is developed from experience and increased perceptual awareness. This leads to the process of making clinical judgements as an internalized process and builds upon Marks-Maran's (1995) assertion that 'models of nursing are tools by which nurses practise, reflect on that practice, change, if necessary, and improve future practice'.

Eliciting constructs may be undertaken using a number of procedures, the simplest being to listen to a subject's conversation, read their essays or listen to their poetry. However, not all constructs are symbolized by words, some are conveyed non-verbally in the form of facial expression or body posture or are manifested in art or music.

Summary

It is suggested that personal construct theory not only has the potential as a model for nursing, but also for complementary therapies, thus allowing complementary therapies or procedures from the therapies and nursing to blend, promoting a seamless integration that enables nurses to offer a wider range of interventions in their nursing care. By coming together in a therapeutic relationship using personal construct theory, it is possible for nurses to enhance the process of healing which is an integral part of nursing care.

REFERENCES

Benner P 1984 From novice to expert: excellence and power in clinical nursing practice. Addison-Wesley, Menlo Park, CA

Boschma G 1994 The meaning of holism in nursing: historical shifts in holistic nursing ideas. Public Health Nursing 11 (5): 324–330

Buckle J 1993 When is holism not complementary. British Journal of Nursing, 2 (15): 744–745

Fulder S 1996 The handbook of alternative and complementary medicine: the essential health companion. Vermilion, London

Ham-Ying S 1993 Analysis of the concept of holism within the context of nursing. British Journal of Nursing 2 (15): 771–775

Henderson V 1966 The nature of nursing. Collier Macmillan, London

Kelly G 1955 The psychology of personal constructs, Vol 1. Norton, New York

Kershaw B 1992 Nursing models: the self-image of the nurse. In: Jolley M Brykczynska G (eds) Nursing care: the challenge to change. Arnold, London

Korbet L , Folan M 1990 Coming of age in nursing. Nursing and Health Care 11 (6): 309–312

Levine M 1971 Holistic nursing. Nursing Clinics of North America 6 (2): 253–264

Levine M 1983 Introduction to clinical nursing. Davis, Philadelphia

Marks-Maran D 1995 Procrustes in the ward: fitting people into models. In: Jolley M, Bryczynska G (eds) Nursing beyond tradition and conflict. Mosby, London

Miccozzi M S 1996 Characteristics of complementary and alternative medicine. In: Fundamentals of complementary and alternative medicine. Churchill Livingstone, Edinburgh

Neuman B 1974 The Betty Neuman health care systems model: a total person approach to patient problems. In: Riehl J Roy C (eds) Conceptual models for nursing practice. Appleton-Century-Crofts, New York

Neuman B 1982 The Neuman systems model: application to nursing education and practice. Appleton-Century-Crofts, New York

Newbeck I Rowe D 1986 Going the whole way. Nursing Times February 19: 24–25

Orem D 1985 Nursing: concepts of practice. McGraw-Hill, New York

Pearson A Vaughan B 1986 Nursing models for practice. Heinemann, London

Rogers M 1970 The theoretical basis of nursing. Davis, Philadelphia

Roper N Logan W Tierney A 1985 The elements of nursing. Churchill Livingstone, Edinburgh

Roy C 1974 The Roy adaptation model. In: Riehl J Roy C (eds) Conceptual models for nursing practice. Appleton-Century-Crofts, New York

Roy C 1984 Introduction to nursing: an adaptation model. Prentice-Hall, Englewood Cliffs

Sharma U 1994 The equation of responsibility. In: Budd S Sharma U (eds) The healing bond. Routledge, London

Todd B 1990 Holistic nursing: a new paradigm for practice. NSNA/Imprint September/October: 75–80

Trevelyan J Booth B 1994 Complementary medicine for nurses, midwives and health visitors. Macmillan Press, London

Vincent C Furnham A 1997 Complementary medicine: a research perspective. John Wiley, London

Watson J 1979 The philosophy and science of caring. Little Brown, Boston

SECTION 2

Approaches to healing

10 Sacred space – right relationship in health and healing: not just what we do but who we are

Stephen G Wright   Jean Sayre-Adams

'Sacred or secular, what is the difference?
If every atom inside our bodies was once a star,
Then it is all sacred
And all secular
At the same time.'   Gretel Erhlich (1987)

INTRODUCTION

Much of the current writing, research and practice in the field of the complementary therapies have leaned more and more towards the 'health technology' perspective. The accelerating drive to integrate complementary therapies into mainstream or orthodox health care has occurred in parallel with the pressure to regularize their scientific and research basis (FIM 1998). The trend is reinforced by the policy demands for evidence-based medicine at every level of the health care system, and shored up by fears of litigation and pressures to control costs. A picture emerges more and more of the complementary therapies, once greeted with near derision and hostility from the medical establishment, being integrated as treatments like any other. The aromatherapy oil or the reflexology session is thereby deemed to be subject to the same rigorous rules of scientific scrutiny and diagnostic application as any other medicine. Thus, integration in this view means the therapy must stand up to scientific standards if it is to be accepted, and can then be used as a treatment, a health technology intervention like any other. A diagnosis is made, and appropriate treatment can now be prescribed based on the evidence.

It is difficult to gainsay this approach. Like motherhood and apple pie, science, research and evidence are so self-evidently good that to question them is considered anarchic, outrageous or unprofessional.

Certainly, where public safety is concerned, it would seem reasonable to subject the complementary therapies to the same rigorous scrutiny and controls as any other medical intervention. A full discussion of the limitations of the scientific and medical models is beyond the scope of this chapter, and the authors are not advocating a free-for-all which exposes patients and clients to all manner of charlatanism and quackery (a not uncommon feature of the complementary *and* orthodox territories when viewed historically). It is right to be concerned with issues of public safety and the testing of all health care techniques. However, it does seem appropriate to reflect upon why so many patients and practitioners turned to the complementary therapies in the first place. It seems that seekers are looking for more than cures for illness (Woodham & Peters 1998). People also seek time, personal attention, involvement in their care and treatment, understanding (and learning from) the disease process, comfort, reassurance, a sense of healing and wholeness. These and other features suggest that people have made use of the complementary therapies for more than a cure for an illness. Is there a risk that the 'more' which people seek can be lost if the therapies are fully integrated into the symptoms–diagnosis–treatment model? Will the complementary therapies make much difference to people's health if they become another line on the treatment sheet?

Furthermore, the linear approach of the medical model – therapist or clinician treats, patient receives – is somewhat antagonistic to the much espoused view that the complementary therapies fit into a holistic health view. Holism, in this sense, is more than seeing people as an accretion of biological, social, psychological and spiritual systems. Holism, rooted in concepts derived from quantum physics and the post-Einsteinian thinkers (Bohm 1973, Talbot 1991) suggests that everything is interconnected. In this model, it is not possible to see the patient as a totally separate entity from the clinician or therapist. That which affects one, at some level affects the other.

HOLISM

Holism is much more than the limited attempts at description which often appear in health care literature or in common parlance. These often amount to just another form of reductionism. Holism is sometimes thought of as giving total care to the patient's biopsychosocial needs. Latterly it has become fashionable to add spiritual needs as well. Holism is not about biopsychosociospiritual care! Rather, it encourages us to think of human beings as part of the universe which is a dynamic web of interconnected and interrelated events, none of which function in isolation. Bohm (1973) writes that, 'There has been too little emphasis on what is, in our view, the most fundamentally different new feature of all, i.e. the intimate interconnectedness of different systems that are not in spatial contact ... the parts are seen to be in immediate connection, in which their dynamical relationships depend, in an irreducible way, on the state of the whole system (and indeed on that broader system in which they are contained, extending ultimately and in principle to the entire universe.) Thus one is led to a new notion of unbroken wholeness which denies the classical idea of analysability of the world into separate and independently existing parts.' Holism asks us to reach out beyond our limited definitions of what people are, passed down in biological, medical, sociological and psychological models. It also leads us into the view that healer and patient can no longer be seen as separate entities when healing is being sought. We are all caught up in the healing process together. Martha Rogers (1970) in her nursing theory of 'unitary human beings', was one of the first to bring this new paradigm into a nursing and health care context.

This can be illuminated in the work of Young (1995) who writes, 'There can be a moment in healing when there is perfect balance and all distinction ... between wounded and healer disappears. It is at this moment that something else can enter and both are transported to a place of mystery. Part of us yearns to return to that place because it is here that we are made whole.' This sense of participating together in a healing process, where distinctions merge, offers us a perspective on the holistic nature of healing. It differs markedly from the traditional paradigm that healing concerns only what one person does to another, i.e. injects a drug, applies a treatment etc. In the holistic sense, healing takes place as much with the involvement of the healer as the patient, and beyond, to take account of the whole healing context which in turn is influenced by all that is.

If healing emerges through the conscious participation of both healer and patient and the whole environment (where, in a holistic sense, there is in fact no healer, or patient or environment, but an interconnected web of participation) then this begs some questions of the way in which the healer participates. Two key issues can be briefly considered here. The first concerns the nature of consciousness, the second the nature of the healing relationship.

CONSCIOUSNESS

Health professionals have often been trained to use the term 'state of consciousness' to describe a continuum from 'normal' behaviour to pathological or altered states varying from drug manipulation to psychotic states, from metabolic derangement to post-traumatic head injuries (Dossey et al 1988). However, much of cutting edge science in the field of consciousness research is illuminating how very limited this view is. Newman (1986) theorizes that true health occurs only as our consciousness expands. An increasing body of evidence is pointing to the non-locality of consciousness (Dossey 1993, 1997); in other words, consciousness is not just about what we loosely consider taking place in the 'mind' with thought, dreams and ideas. It actually impacts upon our bodies and the wider world in infinitely more complex ways than has hitherto been considered or researched. The work of Pert (1997) for example, working in the field of psychoneuroimmunology is showing how our emotions can affect the physical state of the body, while Benson (1975) and others have documented the non-local possibilities of healing, for example through prayer, which do not require the healer to be in the physical presence of the patient. Thus, what these and other studies and theorists are pointing to is a greatly expanded understanding of the nature of consciousness than has generally been considered in orthodox health care, and which has enormous implications for human well-being in the future.

One thing all this points to is the possibility that the interventions which therapists use in seeking the healing of another may only be part of the story. Indeed they may turn out to be only a bit part of the grand drama that is the healing process. It may be that all our treatments and potions are less about biological effects on bodies, than something that switches the consciousness of the patient into mobilizing the body's molecular energy and other resources into healing itself. Such a scenario can be extended into the possibility that healing can emerge when all treatments fall away, and the presence of the two in the search for healing is enough to create the space in which healing emerges.

HEALING RELATIONSHIPS

If healing is triggered in the relationship between patient and healer, interacting in the total environment, and consciously participating in healing, then this begs some questions about the quality of that relationship. Why do not all therapist–patient relationships work (in the sense of 'working' as producing a successful healing or curing outcome, an expansion of consciousness and awareness, a feeling of becoming more whole as a person, feeling better, even though dying)? This seems to depend upon the depth of the 'right relationship'.

To enter right relationship with others it is not possible to bypass the emotional work upon ourselves, to enter into right relationship with ourselves. In other words our potential in the healing process is greatly enhanced when we have taken a long hard look at who we are, what makes us 'tick' and how we are in the world. We may realize that such work is unending, a continuous, slow cooking of the psyche as we mature, experience and perhaps actively work on deepening our awareness of who we are and why we are here. Such work, spiritual work, is not undertaken by many. Large numbers of people remain stuck in a particular way of being that may remain very little changed until they die. The person who seeks to be a true healer of others knows that this is not possible without healing themselves – coming home to who they really are, healing old wounds, letting go of old agendas about power and control. Thus we come into full consciousness of ourselves in order to participate fully and consciously in healing. Right relationship therefore begins with ourselves.

As we enter into a healing right relationship with another, it is characterized by a 'harmonious, balanced, attentive, action-orientated way of being in the world. It is built on values of respect and reverence for persons and the whole of creation, seeking to be in relationship with them in patterns which are loving, supportive, available and not hooked on models of power, control, and abuse. It seeks to nourish and aid others to choose and pursue their own life path, to make right choices that are equally loving and nourishing for them, without imposing our will or world-view upon them. Indeed in right relationship, there is no us and them, no separation, but an acknowledgement of the inescapable interconnectedness of all life, all relationships, all creation' (Wright & Sayre-Adams 2000). In right relationship we find the qualities of trust, faith, honesty, integrity are embedded in the healing process which healer and patient enter. Indeed, trust and a belief in the healer, considering the studies on consciousness cited above, appear to be significant factors in triggering the healing response, as is the belief in the patients themselves that they can heal. The interplay of consciousness between healer and patient, bonded in right relationship, is the milieu in which healing emerges. The therapies and treatments may be just gateways through which this process can walk, the hooks of 'doing' to allow 'being' and healing to happen.

Thus in right relationship, we do not so much help others, but become available and centred in ourselves in ways which allow others to help and heal themselves. If right relationship is the medium for healing, nourished by the conscious participation of both parties in the whole healing context, then how is this created? Perhaps more accurately, how is it co-created, for in a holistic sense as has been suggested, this is not the linear model of healer doing unto patient.

SACRED SPACE

Coming into right relationship is a sacred act. Entering the place of stillness in ourselves, set apart momentarily from what we come to realize are the trivia of life where we can discover our true being, indeed just 'be', we can re-connect with our senses and return to the world to participate fully and safely in all its beauty and tragedy.

Making time for stillness helps us to come home to ourselves, and discover that home is sacred. This is the focus of spiritual teachings for millennia. The word sacred has its origins in the Latin 'sacrare' to consecrate or make holy. It is deeply imbued with religious and spiritual connotations – concerning rituals and practices associated with our desire to understand and connect with the divine such as sacred music or writings. The Bible, the Qur'an, the Upanishads are sacred texts. Much of the finest music, prose and poetry across the generations has been inspired by and sought to represent the sacred. Sacred space, and its instruments – beauty, stillness, music and so on – inspires and uplifts us. It 'fills us with awe, with joy, with wellbeing, that which adds meaning to our lives' (Angwin 1998). Whether we adopt a theistic or atheistic world view does not matter. The sacred concerns reverence for all of life, for rituals and places that connect us to that deep core in our being that we have called the Self, God, the Absolute, the One. Sacred space can be places where we feel that connection more strongly than in others, where there is 'a construction in the imagination that affirms the independence of the holy' (Lane 1988). Sacred space is the instrument of our unfolding spirituality, the tool to do the work; it is also the realized outcome as we discover the sacred in all things, including ourselves.

Can we 'make' sacred space? It is possible to set up an altar in our office, build a shrine in our garden or create a certain ceremony or ritual, but these do not become sacred in themselves. Things become sacred because of the significance and reverence with which we hold them. They form part of a sacred act because of the consciousness from ourselves with which we imbue them, the beliefs and feelings we attach to them. The sacred can therefore be 'out there' in terms of special places or actions – a religious service, a particularly beautiful forest, landscape, or special building.

However, to 'create' sacred space is at another level a contradiction in terms. If everything is part of the whole and interconnected, then everything is sacred. All that changes is our awareness of it. Thus we do not so much 'make' sacred space, insofar as we may change the physical environment in some way, as participate in it – and participate by shifting our awareness, our consciousness toward the sacred. Sacred space is thus both internal and external, within us and beyond, it is 'here' already eternally present, all we have to do is 'tune in' to it, become aware of it, realize it. The sacred is all around us and in each one of us; we do not so much create sacred space as co-create with it, come to an awareness of it, know it, pay attention to it and participate mindfully in it.

Sacred space is a place where wonder can be revealed, where the 'divine or the supernatural can be glimpsed or experienced, where we can get in touch with that which is larger than ourselves' (Lane 1988).

Getting in touch with sacred space requires active intention and having become aware of its possibility, it then allows us to work with it, to enhance healing environments, to have reverence for all that is taking place in our immediate world and the wider world around us – respect for the planet, action for healing. In opening to the sacred, the intention is to move beyond reverence into action, compassionate action. Sacred space is a place of spiritual work, where the consciousness and power of ourselves and the universe engage in a wondrous interplay that seeks to set all around it in right relationship, to re-collect into wholeness and thereby heal.

Every healing and caring act is a sacred act. In the work world of most carers, replete with a myriad distractions and pressures, the sense of the sacred has been almost completely lost. A few hardy souls may have the strength to integrate it quietly into their work, but for most, if the sacred or spirituality are mentioned at all, they are the subject of scepticism, ridicule or embarrassment. Caught in the struggle of doing the work, we find it hard to stand back from it and take a wider view. Healing and caring still happen, but in ways that are stunted, their potential unfulfilled because right relationships in all parts of the caring context are not fully present. For the healing potential to be fully realized, it requires right relationship not only of the carer or healer with themselves, but also with patients and clients, with teams and colleagues, with wider organizations and the whole healing context.

When we examine the levels of abuse, stress and burnout in many health care settings (Wright & Sayre-Adams 2000), it may be seen as something of wonder that healing emerges at all in the face of such seemingly overwhelming odds of inhospitable clinics and workplaces, disharmonious teams, dysfunctional organizations and the personal baggage we carry with us which stunts our own growth and potential participation in healing. Sacred space does not end at the doors of the sick person's bedroom, the clinic or nursing home, or the hospital ward. It pervades everything, and is potentially available to us in all places and at all times.

The potential of the sacred is enhanced when we wake up to it, when we seek to work with it and hold it in our everyday lives. Its power is unleashed when we seek to create certain spaces that shift our consciousness of the presence of the sacred. It is made fully manifest when we are spurred to action in the world not in the narrow confines of our own goals and ambitions, but to being available as conscious participants, playmates of the sacred, aiding its full realization in every caring moment, every action no matter how mundane or profound. When we are in right relationship with ourselves, the effects ricochet down and out into all our relationships. When we are in right relationship with ourselves, we discover the sacred space that is within. In that discovery comes the realization that what is within is also beyond us – as above, so below. Attuning to the sacred within, we find it in everything as well. Thus grounded and centred in our own being, our own sacredness, we become available for the sacred to radiate into all aspects of our lives, not least our caring and healing work. Thus, we do not so much create sacred space, as become and be it. Who we are is the sacred. Who we are is the healer. We are the sacred space.

Whatever complementary therapy we use may thus be less important than the way we use it. Who we are in the co-creation of healing may be as significant, if not more so, than any therapy we offer.

There is a Sufi saying that 'You think that by understanding one, you can understand two, for one and one is two. But to understand two, you must first understand "and".' It is in the space between, the sacred space, the place of 'and' where we connect. In connection lies right relationship. In right relationship lies the sacred space of healing.

REFERENCES

Angwin R 1998 Creating sacred space. Positive Health Dec/Jan: 6–7

Benson H 1996 Timeless healing. Schuster, London

Bohm D 1973 Quantum theory as an indication of a new order in physics; implicate and explicate order in physical law. Foundation of Physics 3: 139–168

Dossey L 1993 Healing words. Harper, San Francisco

Dossey L 1997 The forces of healing; reflections on energy, consciousness and the beef stroganoff principle. Alternative Therapies in Health and Medicine 3 (5): 8–14

Dossey B Keegan L Guzetta C Kolkmeier L 1988 Holistic nursing: a handbook for practice. Aspen, Gaithersburg, MD

Erhlich G 1987 Landscape. In: Sullivan C (ed) The legacy of light. Knopf, New York

Foundation for Integrated Medicine (FIM) 1998 Integrated healthcare: a way forward for the next five years? FIM, London

Lane B C 1988 Landscapes of the sacred. Paulist, New York

Newman M 1986 Health as expanding consciousness. Mosby, St Louis

Pert C 1997 Molecules of emotion. Scribner, New York

Rogers M E 1970 An introduction to the theoretical basis for nursing. Davies, Philadelphia

Talbot M 1991 The holographic universe. Harper Collins, New York

Woodham A Peters D 1998 The encyclopaedia of complementary medicine. Dorling Kindersley, London

Wright S G Sayre-Adams J 2000 Sacred space – right relationship and spirituality in healthcare. Churchill Livingstone, Edinburgh

Young M 1995 In: Forder J Forder E (eds) The light within. Usha, Dent

11 Shamanism

Mike Money

INTRODUCTION

When European explorers first saw shamanic healing they tended to be dismissive (Mitrani 1992). Today, after 200 years of comparative neglect (Atkinson 1992) there has been a resurgence of interest and a growing recognition that shamanism may offer profound insights into many contemporary issues in health and healing. With a wide geographical distribution and a long history shamanism may reconnect us with some elements essential to understanding the human condition.

WHAT IS SHAMANISM?

Shamanism seems to be at least 30 000 years old and to be found in almost all human cultures. It may well be one of the earliest characteristically human activities and have influenced all human societies and belief systems. For example, what we call witchcraft may have been a form of European shamanism. The story of Jacob and the angel may be a tale of shamanic initiation. Work on Romani shamanism is forthcoming (Lee 2000). Added to this, modern interpretations of shamanic practice have emerged using such labels as 'shamanistic' 'neo-shamanic' or 'urban shamanism' (e.g Roth 1990, Krippner & Welch 1992)).

Shamanism connects with many modern issues in health and healing. Although not a religion, it is certainly a spiritual tradition, and may enable us to discuss the spiritual dimension to health in nonsectarian language. Shamanism also contains a powerful ecological perspective. Now that Westerners are at last realizing that what we do to the planet, the planet eventually does back to us, that perspective is highly appropriate. Shamanism places great emphasis on the tribal connection – on relationships within and between communities. With our increasingly fragmented social structure, that may be a message we need to hear again. Shamanism addresses those key moments in our lives when we move from one role to another – marriage, parenthood, death – which anthropologists call *rites of passage*. Shamanism addresses issues of personal change and growth, and the integration of growth and change into the totality of one's life. Illness and the therapeutic moment are particularly powerful examples of such change.

Shamanic practice suggests that there are several possible states of human consciousness, and that 'normal' waking consciousness is not the only one worth having. Shamans learn to make a voluntary and controlled transition to another state of conscious awareness which Harner (1990) calls the Shamanic State of Consciousness. Within this state, the shaman has access to knowledge, insights and information which they cannot normally command. A useful analogy is that of driving a car. There is no such thing as the one right gear, only the right gear relative to the specifics of the driving task. So for the shaman, the right state of consciousness is the appropriate one for the task in hand, and shamans will engage different states of consciousness using a variety of techniques, including dancing, drumming, chanting and dreaming. As part of this process, shamans often experience a restructuring of their own identity and of their relationship with the rest of the cosmos.

Mircea Eliade's (1964) influential book on shamanism described it as 'archaic techniques of ecstasy'. That word 'ecstasy' can mislead, for shamanic practice is characterized by control (Kressing 1997) rather than drug-induced euphoria. A restriction upon some Western approaches to healing is the assumption that only one state of consciousness is valid or appropriate, and that therefore only one sort of knowledge is worthwhile. Those concerned with the epistemological basis of complementary therapies may find this point important.

It is difficult to encapsulate the shamanic experience and its healing implications within a small compass. However, shamanism is essentially about practice, and it is possible to indicate those elements of shamanic practice which may be or become relevant to current issues in health and healing.

WHY IS SHAMANISM RELEVANT TO HEALING?

Shamanic principles may interest anyone engaged in the healing enterprise. As Harner (1996) observes: 'Healing is one of the key functions the shaman fulfils in most communities worldwide' (p 90). We should recognize healing enterprise as going beyond those issues normally addressed as part of physical health. There are good grounds for exploring shamanism as the basis for a new approach to mental health and its promotion, which does not seem readily addressed by conventional biomedical models. It may be that people working in the complementary area are well-placed to insert such insights as may be appropriate into their own practice.

But it is principles rather than specifics that are addressed here. A pick-and-mix approach to the shamanic tradition is at best disorientating and at worst confusing to client and practitioner alike. Practices that are familiar and appropriate in one culture could easily be phony or frightening if transplanted to another, and would bring no therapeutic benefit. The principles, however, may well be portable, and may help us reconstruct or rediscover a tradition of our own. This chapter explores some of the reasons this may be so, and considers some possible implications particularly for practitioners of complementary therapies. Some of these implications have been explored previously by the author (Money 1997).

Understanding and facilitating personal change and growth

As writers on shamanism (e.g. Eliade 1964) point out, the process of becoming a shaman can be painful. At best it is attended by illness or privation, at the worst by terrifying images of dismemberment and death. Apprentice shamans are said to experience descent into the realm of demons, their bodies are torn apart and their bones scattered. These are painful experiences. But after dismembering comes its opposite – re-membering. The mutilated body is reconstructed; the terrifying experiences are interpreted within a framework that makes them significant and worthwhile; they are seen as the price to be paid for insights which will energize the individual for the rest of their life. The price is paid gladly, whether chosen or not.

Illness and change are seldom as dramatic as this but they are intimately connected and people experiencing them can be helped by those who have already undergone such an experience. Jung is said to have observed that only the wounded healer can heal. Change and transformation are intrinsic to the shamanic experience and shamanic principles may thus be relevant to negotiating the changes of illness. For example, Jilek (e.g. 1992) has published considerable work on the revival of shamanic dance amongst the Salish Indians. The Salish Spirit Dance has been reconstructed as a healing ceremony, and Jilek regards it as therapeutically effective. Another Native American healing ritual – the Sun Dance – has been positively evaluated by Wong (1996). The shamanic tradition emphasizes illness and healing as important and educational times of change, and that methods of marking, facilitating and even celebrating such change may be of great significance to the healing process. Shamanic healing necessitates exploring the meaning of illness for a particular person, and the negotiation of intervention and outcome. This approach closely mirrors the holistic healing paradigm employed by many complementary practitioners.

A repository of rites of passage

Knowing when adulthood has been reached is not as easy as it used to be. The idea that one is an adult at 21 is obsolete and we now acquire different aspects of adult status at different ages. This fluidity is also true for other great life landmarks – birth, naming, puberty, marriage, parenthood, grand-parenthood. Our present lack of such meaningful rites may give rise to doubts about identity and adult status, and may impel young people – denied rituals sanctioned by society – to invent their own. A home-grown initiation may be needlessly dangerous or lack the framework of guidance, meaning and protection that accompanies the transition to adult status in shamanic cultures (e.g. Halifax 1979). The shamanic tradition strongly suggests the need to regenerate or reinvent rites of passage, and we may fail our children if we do not. Baker's (1992) work on childbirth is an instructive example of how a rite of passage can be developed. Roth's (1990) moving account of her own father's dying is another lucid example. Such rituals enable us to conceptualize the changes we experience, they may bind together those who experience them and they may be intimately bound up with our self-esteem and sense of identity – essential to the maintenance of personal health.

A positive perspective on death and dying

It has been suggested that the present is a good time for shamanic practice because we are already dismembered. In comparison with members of traditional cultures, people in the West have no tribe or extended family to belong to, no rites of passage to confirm us as adults, no new name to reflect key events in our lives, no totem society to which we belong, little shared ritual other than the vicarious participation offered by television when a royal wedding is enacted. No more is there a shared mythology uniting the sacred and the profane, the mundane with the eternal. In comparison with inhabitants of traditional cultures, even on a good day, we are dismembered. Then add illness, pain, anxiety or distress.

It is a common experience when ill to search for meaning, to ask why this experience is being undergone, to seek its significance. Yet while biomedicine may be excellent at addressing some of our ills, it is poor at exploring the purpose and meaning of illness, dying and death. From the shamanic perspective these are immensely important learning experiences, and have long been recognized within the shamanistic tradition as positive and salutogenic. As Buckley (1994) writes, 'When viewed positively, death becomes an ally, offering the incentive and potential for maximising a meaningful existence in this life as we experience it now' (p 41).

The shamanic perspective does not mean to minimize the pain and distress of those who are ill or dying, or that of their relatives. But approaching illness or death as one further rite of passage, one more learning opportunity, one more window through which insight may be glimpsed, could be profoundly salutogenic. It would certainly contrast with the experiences some have had within the conventional system. There may well be scope here for practitioners of complementary therapies.

Imagery and healing

Imagery has long been a part of shamanic therapeutics. As Achterberg (1985) powerfully demonstrated, shamanism is above all the medicine of the imagination. That is not to say, however, that it is imaginary medicine. Shamanic healing frequently entails the use of positive, familiar and encouraging imagery to precipitate or facilitate the healing process (Crohn 1995). Clients are encouraged to form as concrete an image of their illness as they can, and this image is often used to identify the problem and to initiate the healing process. A vivid account illustrating this process in given by Mehl-Madrona (1997).

What is noteworthy is a steady accumulation of evidence within the Western tradition strongly suggesting that imagery (a broader term than the *visualization* sometimes employed) has a very powerful contribution to make to the healing process. In 1978, Simenton et al published research showing that visual imagery, when coupled with more orthodox approaches such as surgery or radiotherapy, produced strikingly better results than the orthodox alone. They described how one patient whose throat cancer was successfully addressed transferred the techniques to his other problems of arthritis and impotence. Achterberg (1985), and more recently Graham (1995), also provide strong evidence for the role of imagery in healing. Appropriate imagery seems central to the effective use of methods such as biofeedback; recent research in the developing field of psychoneuroimmunology also indicates how this might be understood biologically. It has been suggested (Harner & Tryon 1996) that shamanic interventions may have positive psychological effects and positive consequences for immune function. The therapeutic use of imagery is thus an area of contact between shamanic and more orthodox approaches to healing. Indeed, it is possible that the use of the shamanic perspective might help us to develop a further integration of the two (Money 1996a) within a broader healing paradigm.

There are several relevant points here for practitioners of complementary therapies. The first two are already implicit in what has been said, that the use of a client's imagery may be valuable in identifying their own conceptualization of the problem and that the use of positive imagery may promote healing. But shamanic healers are also very careful to create and maintain an environment charged with positive and encouraging imagery, both internal (in terms of the way they listen and speak to their client) and external (in how they structure the healing environment in both physical and social dimensions). It is possible to ask how many hospital settings reflect the intentional creation of a physical environment that is positive and encouraging.

The promotion of mental health

The promotion of health is not the same as the treatment of illness. Black is not white, up is not down, and health is not illness. Therefore mental health is not mental illness. Working for mental health is not the same thing as screening for, educating about, or treating mental illness, although all those activities may be a necessary but not sufficient precondition for the promotion of mental health. Although complementary therapy, being therapy, will usually address a problem or an issue, it also has a potential, perhaps not fully realized, for the promotion of mental health.

There are many factors contributing to health, and therefore many contributing to mental health. Previous papers have attempted to explore the potential of shamanic approaches to mental health (Money 1993, 1994) and have argued (Money 1996b) that these approaches can be brought together under five categories or dimensions – the individual, the interpersonal, the power locus, the environmental and the therapeutic. Complementary therapies have the potential to contribute positively to at least three of these. In the case of power locus, there is considerable evidence (e.g. Dossey 1991) that people who feel in control of their own lives and who make their own decisions enjoy better health and longer lives than those who do not. Being ill may in itself be a negation of these features, but the ability to exercise choice of therapy – whether orthodox or complementary – must be positive. If therapy is delivered in a way that acknowledges the person at the other end of the process, then so much the better; the interpersonal is then also addressed. A criticism sometimes heard of biomedicine is that the person – as opposed to the condition – may sometimes be neglected. Clearly, if the remedy is effective then the removal of anxiety about pain, illness and the availability of the treatment of choice will also be therapeutic.

It will be understood, however, that distinguishing between physical and mental health is in fact fruitless. Human beings are one entity and the promotion of health must ultimately address all aspects of our being. Mental health promotion can be forgotten, or relegated to the pathological, so this section's heading serves to remind us of a neglected domain. But what has been said about promoting mental health here is true for health per se. Shamanic perspectives suggest that people need a clear sense of their own identity; that they need frequent and positive contact with family, friends and the wider community; that they need to make their own decisions and feel in charge of their own lives; that they need contact with the wider natural world; and that they need appropriate and compassionate healing when they are ill. A key element in this is our relationship with the rest of the natural world, and the insight that flows from an ecological perspective.

Ecological insight, health and healing

Since the 1960s, ecological issues have moved from minority to mainstream. It is now accepted that not only do we live in the world but the world lives in us – that global health and human health are inseparable. This perception has always been part of the shamanic tradition, and shamans have served as advocates of the ecosystem at their particular spot on the planet (White 1995, Reichel-Dolmatoff 1997). We now share this perspective and understand that clean air, clean water, fresh food and space to enjoy them are essential to all aspects of our well-being. Complementary practitioners are probably sympathetic to this position and the point requires no labouring.

An ecological perspective links the promotion of human health to the maintenance of a healthy planet. This implies that biodiversity, the opportunity to walk in the mountains without hearing traffic, to stroll through a forest without hearing a chainsaw, to interact with wild animals rather than pampered pets, to wade along a river bed, are all central to our health. Whether we categorize well-being as physical, emotional, mental, or spiritual is in the end arbitrary. It may be argued that the source of many health problems is what Berman (1981) has termed *disenchantment*; a loss of perception of meaning and purpose in the rest of the universe. The therapy is re-enchantment: the conversion of depression into happiness, of inertia into ecstasy. This is the essence of shamanic practice. Interesting work has been carried out here by Ingerman (1991), who has applied the shamanic technique of soul retrieval to a variety of emotional and physical diseases. The ultimate point is that whatever increases a person's feelings of happiness, worth and competence will benefit their whole health.

SUMMARY

It was argued earlier that the focus of this chapter was principles not practice. What might practitioners of complementary therapy gain from shamanic principles?

- Shamanic principles can illuminate elements of current practice, indicate where practice might be developed or enhanced, suggest new directions for research and serve as a framework within which new and existing therapies can be integrated.

- Shamanic principles place the person and their inner world rather than the technology at the heart of the healing enterprise, and define well-being in terms of personal wholeness and integration. The rediscovery of such a healing system strongly supports the complementary practitioner's principle of focusing on whole people rather than clinically-defined patients.

- Recent research suggests that shamanic practice is congruent with emerging holistic perspectives of health, and psychoneuroimmunology in particular seems to endorse the shaman's focus on the images of the client's inner world. One consequence would be the intentional creation of positive and encouraging imagery at every point in the healing process, including physical setting and the language of interaction.

- The validation of more than one sort of knowledge may be reassuring to complementary practitioners as it confirms the principle that healing systems do not have to be wholly compatible with Western biomedicine in order to be worthwhile.

- Shamanic principles reaffirm the significance of a spiritual dimension to healing.

To conclude, it may well be that the renaissance of interest in shamanism may be especially relevant and timely to practitioners of complementary therapies, who may be particularly well placed to participate in our growing understanding of the healing potential of shamanism.

REFERENCES

Achterberg J 1985 Imagery and healing – shamanism and modern medicine. Shambhala, Boston

Baker J P 1992 The shamanic dimensions of childbirth. Pre- and Peri-Natal Psychology Journal 7: 1

Berman M 1981 The re-enchantment of the world. Cornell University Press, Ithaca

Buckley E 1994 The shamanic path to mental health: death as an ally. In: Trent D R Reed C (eds) Promotion of mental health, Vol 3. Avebury, Aldershot

Crohn B 1995 A shamanic approach to surviving cancer. Shaman's Drum 37: 49–51

Dossey L 1991 Healing breakthroughs. Piatkus, London

Eliade M 1964 Shamanism – archaic techniques of ecstasy. Arcana, London

Graham H 1995 A picture of health – how to use guided imagery for self-healing and personal growth. Piatkus, London

Harner M 1990 The way of the shaman, 3rd edn. Harper, San Francisco

Harner S Tryon W W 1996 Psychological and immunological responses to shamanic journeying with drumming. Shaman 4: 1–2

Halifax J 1979 Shamanic voices. Arkana, London

Kressing F 1997 Candidates for a theory of shamanism. A systematic survey of recent research results from Eurasia and Native America. Shaman 5: 2

Krippner S Welch P 1992 Spiritual dimensions of healing – from native shamanism to contemporary health care. Irvington, New York

Lee P J 2000 We borrow the earth – the art and life of a gypsy healer. Thorsons, London (in press)

Mehl-Madrona L 1997 Coyote medicine – lessons from Native American healing. Rider, London

Money M C 1993 The shamanic path to mental health promotion. In: Trent D R Reed C (eds) Promotion of mental health, Vol 2. Avebury, Aldershot

Money M C 1994 Following the shamanic path to mental health promotion. In: Trent D R Reed C (eds) Promotion of mental health, Vol 3. Avebury, Aldershot

Money M C 1996a Shamanism as a healing paradigm. Occasional paper, Institute for Health, Liverpool John Moores University, Liverpool

Money M C 1996b Dimensions of positive mental health. Occasional paper, Institute for Health, Liverpool John Moores University, Liverpool

Money M C 1997 Shamanism and complementary therapy. Complementary Therapies in Nursing and Midwifery

Roth G 1990 Maps to ecstasy – teachings of an urban shaman. Mandala, London

Simenton O C Matthews-Simenton S Creighton J 1978 Getting well again. Tarcher, Los Angeles

Wong S H 1996 The healing path of the Lakota Sun Dance. Shaman's Drum 43: 49–52

FURTHER READING

Cowan T 1993 Fire in the head – shamanism and the Celtic spirit. Harper, San Francisco

Graham H 1999 Complementary therapies in context – the psychology of healing. Jessica Kingsley, London

Kalweit H 1992 Shamans, healers and medicine men. Shambhala, Boston

Matthews J 1991 Taliesin – shamanism and the bardic mysteries in Britain and Ireland. Aquarian, London

Vitebsky P 1995 The shaman. Macmillan, London

Wolf F A 1991 The eagle's quest. Mandala, London

12 Developing health care environments

Francis C Biley

INTRODUCTION

It was Florence Nightingale, who said, as many nurses are very aware, that the main function of the nurse is to place the patient in the best possible environment for nature to act (Nightingale 1859). The great nursing theorist and academic, Martha Rogers, echoed these words when she asserted that nursing should seek to direct and redirect patterns of interaction between man and his environment for the realization of maximum health potential (Rogers 1970, 1990). However, at present, we almost seem to have forgotten the importance and potential of creating a positive healing environment in hospitals and other health care venues. As Starhawk stated (cited in Venolia 1988), nothing is easier to see than consciousness once we recognize that it is embodied in the forms and structures that we create.

Nursing might be able to realize its healing potential by raising awareness and altering the prevailing consciousness of hospital and healing centre design away from its current, but perhaps misguided, emphasis on functional design and towards the aesthetic. This can be achieved by caring for and manipulating the surroundings to place the patient in the best possible environment for healing.

THE FOCUS OF MODERN NURSING

The focus of modern Western nursing has been, and perhaps still is, the patient, but not in their entirety. Nursing has been either parts- or task-driven. At one time tasks were allocated hierarchically: junior nurses bathed patients and made beds, while only more senior nurses were allowed to take temperatures, blood pressures and do dressings. Today, the nature of the tasks have changed. Today's nurses are allocated small groups of patients, and gone is the ward round handing out 34 Nelson's inhalers to 34 patients every 4 hours. Nurses have become specialized, being experts in diabetes, pressure area or wound care, massage or aromatherapy, reflexology or therapeutic touch. So what has changed? Ten or 20 years ago when care was task-driven, there were specialists in Nelson's inhalers. Today, when care is supposed to be individualized, there are specialists in performing the task of massage, or reflexology or a whole host of other such interventions. Holism is still the dream of a few, yet to be realized by many.

The focus of care is still dominated by the medical model, still dominated by the pursuit of curing, but needs to change. In holism the focus moves away from the patient and towards the environment and the context in which the individual operates in the world.

THE HEALING ENVIRONMENT

Get the environment right and the patient will start to heal themself. When people are ill, in the words of Margo Adair, 'we tend to forget our connection to the earth, to the sky, to each other, to the life that's constantly percolating in and around us. When people forget their connections they wind up feeling drained and isolated. When people remember their connections they become energised, inspired, and feel a part of all that's around us' (Adair 1970). Manipulating the hospital environment means reconnecting with the sky, each other and to life.

There is an old Italian proverb that says, 'Where the sun does not enter, the doctor does'. In the same vein, Norman Cousins stated that 'a hospital is no place for a person who is seriously ill'. But why should that be? Is it because we have focused for too long on just the patient, or parts of the patient, ignoring the environment in which they have to function and become well? It has not always been like that.

Early Greek places of healing, the Asclepian temples, placed great emphasis on surroundings. The temples were built in positions of great beauty so that the patients could enjoy the views, were near natural springs so that the water would be pure and were in raised positions to receive cooling breezes. In the days before most forms of what we now call health care intervention existed, people could do no more than eat good food, rest and sleep, listen to healing music, watch theatrical productions and gain spiritual strength from praying to the gods. More recent history suggests that this kind of approach survived in church buildings, most frequently monasteries, until the early 19th century, when large hospitals began to be built.

When Florence Nightingale made her famous proclamation, quoted earlier, that the environment was critically important, she took steps to ensure that the environment was indeed suitable for healing. One of the first things she did upon her arrival at Scutari was to clean the hospital, whitewash the walls and remove the dead horse from the water supply. Her book, *Notes on Nursing: What it is and What it is Not*, goes further and talks about the importance of having plants, natural light, fresh air, light music and a noise-free environment on the wards (Nightingale 1859).

However, as medical science grew in perceived importance, these positive design elements were gradually removed from the hospital environment. From the mid 19th century onwards, hospital building design began to move away from being temples of healing possessing aesthetic qualities, towards being primarily concerned with function.

Current perspectives in hospital design often concentrate on pragmatism and functionalism, decreeing that expensive machinery should take precedence over ponds and water features, art, gardens, attractive colour schemes and even windows. Why put windows into an intensive care unit if all the patients are unconscious? Regimented care takes place in regimented environments. All that matters about the CAT scanner, X-ray machinery, or birthing table is that they work properly and are easy to clean and repair. The colour of such machinery is unimportant, which is why all machines are a uniform grey, black, or chrome.

Evidence to suggest the need for improvements to the hospital environment

There is a growing body of evidence suggesting that people are paying attention to the environment of care, and that the connection with nature and representations of nature might play a very significant part in healing. Recently built hospitals such as the Chelsea and Westminster and St Mary's Hospital on the Isle of Wight show that there is an ever-increasing concern with the aesthetics of hospital design. There is a large body of evidence to suggest that attention to aesthetics can indeed be healing (Canter & Canter 1979, Carey 1986, Ulrich 1992, Rubin et al 1998). An American architect concerned with hospital design, Roger Ulrich, has found that the display of pictures on walls increases relaxation and provides distraction from other aspects of the environment (Ulrich 1992). Similarly, natural views from hospital windows (of, for example, trees) are thought to have a positive effect on healing (Marcus and Barnes 1995). However, placing pictures on the walls or having windows with nice garden views may be of little use for patients who are lying in bed and who can only look up. Gently illuminated ceiling tiles showing country scenes can very effectively provide distraction. Many hospitals have successfully entered into collaborative relationships with artists and art schemes, and hospital projects are being supported by Arts Councils and organizations such as Arts for Health based in Manchester. For example, Llandough Hospital in Cardiff employs a full-time artist-in-residence who has managed to transform hospital corridors and clinical areas. Similarly, a team of artists were employed to transform the main corridor of a hospital in the north of England, at no more cost than simple redecoration, with large murals and local scenes. The transformation was significant, and it even became a pleasure to walk through the hospital.

SACRED HEALING SITES

In every civilization in the world, there are sacred sites. For example, some Native American Indians believe that health results from being aligned with the many aspects of the cosmos and that to walk in harmony and balance with Mother Earth is to be in a state of health. Illness occurs when we fall out of harmony.

Sacred sites such as healing springs, ceremonial and meditational sites are used in order to restore harmony. The meaning or spirit of place has existed in countless other examples. The Asclepian temples of Epidaurus or Kos, as have already been mentioned, were such places, as were perhaps, the pre-Christian ancient megalithic stone circles and caves and sites such as Glastonbury. Greek philosophy placed great importance on place, with Plato stating that 'some localities have a more marked tendency than others to produce better or worse men'.

With the development of Christianity in the West came the further development of sacred sites, and sacred buildings were erected. In time many of these buildings took on a healing function and were the early temples of healing and early examples of what we now know as modern hospitals. However, modern incarnations of these healing temples worship instrumentalism and modern medicine instead of spiritual values. How can we retain such essential instrumentalism yet at the same time return to being aware of the more spiritual aspects of health and illness?

IMPROVING HOSPITAL DESIGN

We are not always in a position to ensure that the design of hospitals is fully appropriate for optimum patient care and well-being, although well-designed hospital facilities that pay attention to aesthetics do exist. We can, however, decorate that which already exists, e.g. day rooms, ward areas, circulating areas and clinics. There are two major areas where nurses can easily have a significant positive impact on the environment for health care:

- visual environment
- auditory environment.

Visual environment

Pictures can brighten up corridors and rooms, clinics and seating areas (Palmer et al 1999). However, subject matter has been found to be important, and care and thought needs to be taken when choosing such displays. Realistic scenes of land or sea and still life should take preference over portraits, animals and abstract pictures, which may increase confusion and in some instances induce a feeling of being threatened.

This is especially the case for patients who are in an altered state of consciousness, e.g. when recovering from an anaesthetic (Ulrich 1992).

American research has found that patients in intensive care units (ICU) with no view to the outside will occupy ICU beds for longer than patients who can see out of a window (Ulrich 1984). This finding is taken so seriously that in many States it is compulsory to have windows and views from all ICU beds. For those units where this is not possible, specially designed computers run false windows that mimic the passing of the day, where lighting comes up at the beginning of day, clouds pass and the sun sets in the evening. Each of these windows costs in the region of US$9000 and, considering the financial cost of an ICU bed, soon pays back the investment.

The view from the window is important. Particular attention needs to be paid to gardens, with an abundance of flowers being particularly therapeutic. If gardens and outdoor planting cannot be achieved then indoor planting can be a viable alternative. There are considerable benefits to be derived from indoor plants (McDonald 1976), including a reduction in anxiety and a more positive perception of the interior. Not only can they look attractive when well kept, they can perform alternative functions. Plants can 'air scrub', that is clean and purify the air – air quality is an aspect of the environment that Florence Nightingale recognized as being critically important. Indeed, in the 1850s, she stated that it was important to have an aspidistra on the ward. In our present era, when patient empowerment is seen as so important, it has been found that patients who are given control over the care of a plant feel an increase in well-being and self-control (Chang 1978). Mass planting can also alter the acoustics of a room and therefore reduce noise and improve humidification.

The importance of colour

Along with the visuals of two- and three-dimensional art, the use of plants and an awareness of views from windows, whether real or computer-generated, an additional and very powerful form of building manipulation can be achieved with the use of colour. As yet an imprecise art that has pretensions of a science, some aspects of colour theory can be used to great effect. In a ward environment, doors that you would like patients and other users to identify easily, such as to the day room or toilet, should be painted a contrasting colour to the surrounding walls. Similarly, doors that you would not wish these people to frequently use, such as to the clean utility room, should be painted the same colour as the surrounding walls, creating the appearance of continuity (Jacobs and Hustmyer 1974). Such an innovative scheme has been shown to be more effective than even the most obvious sign-posting and can, for example, reduce the incidence of inappropriate wandering in those who are older and have mental health problems.

As mentioned earlier, the colour of hospital machinery is usually black or grey and there is a lack of imagination used in their colour design. However, if you take into account the perceived power of these shades, it is interesting to note that black suggests strength, absorbs and restores energy and protects. It is, however, also associated with primordial darkness, negativity and death. Grey on the other hand represents persistence and spiritual struggle, death and rebirth (Venolia 1988). These colours can be interpreted as powerfully healing, or at the same time destructively negative.

Another aspect of colour that is often overlooked, is the colour of walls. Recommended healing colours are greens, or a mixture of spiritual blue and wise yellow that represents balance, harmony, growth, healing and love. Green is called the master healer and can have central nervous system benefits. Red can be used if stimulation is required, but it is also thought to increase blood pressure, respiration and heart rates, and encourages excitement. Pink is the universal healing colour and is restful and tranquillizing. Yellow can relieve depression and tension, but can have a similar effect to red. It is useful in study areas, particularly if used with blue or violet. Blue can lower blood pressure and is generally restful and can reduce hyperactivity. However, blue rooms are perceived as cooler than warmer coloured rooms (Wood 1984, Venolia 1988). Colour theory should be taken into account in any redecoration scheme.

Auditory environment

Improvement in the auditory environment can have a very positive impact on improving the overall health care environment. Florence Nightingale encouraged nurses to avoid the bustling of crinolines, an early Victorian version of the contemporary proclamation to wear quiet shoes whilst on night duty. She also stated that soothing music was most appropriate for healing the sick and promoting a state of gentle positive contemplation.

Why do we not used piped or background music in hospitals more extensively than we already do? If done properly, gentle background music and the sounds of nature such as waterfalls, streams, or birdsong can have a very positive effect on psychological states and perception of the environment. It can cover up all of those unwanted sounds that seem to travel so far in hospitals. In North America the recommended sound levels for hospitals is 45dBA during the day and 35dBA during the night (USEPA 1974). Putting that into perspective, a quiet conversation is about 45dBA. Yet sound levels above 100dBA have been measured in one hospital department, roughly equivalent to a thundering lorry. A sluice machine can make a noise at the level of about 80dBA and sound levels in incubators have occasionally been found high enough to run the risk of causing long-term hearing loss (Biley 1993). With some creative thought it is possible to achieve a positive auditory background, even in the busiest hospital environment.

CONCLUSION

The environment is an important aspect of healing and an area where nurses can have a positive impact, but is an aspect of care that is generally given low priority, as hospital design seems to follow an industrial model. Attending to the visual environment, in terms of pictures, gardens, indoor planting and colour schemes can make hospitals much more pleasant. Being aware of the auditory environment also brings significant benefits.

In her book, *Sacred Ground to Sacred Space: Visionary Ecology, Perennial Wisdom, Environmental Ritual and Art*, Kryder (1994) stated that 'understanding our sacred ground enables us to discover an alphabet of nature's scripture that we can use to protect and amplify sacred sites and create sacred space. When our consciousness expands to include the sources upon which all things depend, we can tap a healing medicine in even the most devastated environment.'

Nothing is easier to see than consciousness once we recognize that it is embodied in the forms and structures we create and that our current consciousness exists as a functional, instrumentalist state (Starhawk, cited in Venolia 1988). Aesthetics need to be rediscovered in hospital design and concern. Only then can a move be made from the cold sterility of current hospital design into an environment that could be considered much more appropriate. As Nietzsche said, we can use the sublime as the artistic conquest of the horrible. Only then can the adoption of certain complementary therapies and holistic care become maximally effective.

Summary

During the 19th and 20th centuries, as patient care became task-driven, hospital design became primarily concerned with functionalism and instrumentalism. More recently, efforts have been made to improve the environment of care by paying attention to the aesthetics of design. There is evidence to suggest that having a view from a window, being protected from undue noise, having access to gardens, being able to listen to music, view art on the walls and attention to the basic tenets of colour therapy can improve patient outcomes and contribute to the effectiveness of complementary therapies. Only when such environmental issues are addressed can we assert that we are delivering truly holistic care.

REFERENCES

Biley F C 1993 Impact of noise in surgical wards. Surgical Nurse 6: 1, 15–17

Canter D Canter S 1979 Designing for therapeutic environments. John Wiley and Sons, Chichester

Carey D A 1986 Hospice inpatient environments. Van Nostrand Reinhold, New York

Chang B L 1978 Generalized expectancy, situational perceptions and morale. Nursing Research 27: 5, 316–324

Jacobs K Hustmyer F 1974 Effects of four psychological primary colours on GSR, heart rate and respiration rate. Perceptual and Motor Skills 38: 763–766

Kryder R P 1994 Sacred ground to sacred space. Bear and Co, Santa Fe

Marcus C C Barnes M 1995 Gardens in healthcare facilities: uses, therapeutic benefits and design recommendations. The Center for Health Design, Walnut Creek, CA

McDonald E 1976 Plants as therapy. Praeger, New York

Nightingale F 1859 Notes on nursing: what it is and what it is not. Reprinted by Dover Publications, New York, 1969

Palmer J Schanberg L E Kuhn C M 1999 The effect of art on venepuncture induced stress. The Center for Health Design, Walnut Creek, CA

Rogers M E 1970 An introduction to the theoretical basis of nursing. F A Davis, Philadelphia

Rogers M E 1990 Nursing: science of unitary, irreducible, human beings: update 1990. In: Barrett E A M (ed) Visions of Rogers' science-based nursing. National League for Nursing, New York

Rubin H R Owens A J Golden G 1998 An investigation to determine whether the built environment affects patients' medical outcomes. The Center for Health Design, Walnut Creek, CA

Ulrich R S 1984 View though a window may influence recovery from surgery. Science 224: 420–421

Ulrich R S 1992 How design impacts wellness. Healthcare Forum Journal 35: 5, 27–31

USEPA (United States Environmental Protection Agency) 1974 Information on levels of environmental noise requisite to protect public health and welfare with an adequate margin of safety. No. 550/9-74-004. US Government Printing Office, Washington, DC

Venolia C 1988 Healing environments. Celestial Arts, Berkeley

Wood B 1984 The healing power of colour. Destiny, New York

FURTHER READING

General

Cope J 1998 The modern antiquarian. Thorsons, New York

Kryder R P 1994 Sacred ground to sacred space. Bear and Co, Santa Fe

Venolia C 1988 Healing environments. Celestial Arts, Berkeley

Colour

Marberry S O Zagon L 1995 The power of color: creating healthy interior spaces. John Wiley and Sons, Chichester

Sun H Sun D 1993 Color your life. Ballantine, London

Gardens

Gerlach-Spriggs N Kaufman R E Warner S B 1998 Restorative gardens: the healing landscape. Yale University Press, Yale

Hospital Design

Malkin J 1992 Hospital interior architecture. John Wiley & Sons, Chichester

Music

Campbell D 1991 Music physician: for times to come. Theosophical Publishing, London

Goldman J 1991 Healing sounds: the power of harmonics. Element, Dorset

McClellan R 1991 The healing forces of music. Element, Dorset

Nature

Swan J A 1991 The power of place: sacred ground in natural and human environments. Quest, Wheaton

Swan J A 1993 Nature as teacher and healer: how to reawaken your connection with nature. Random House, London

The Arts

Kaye C Blee T 1997 The arts in health care: a palette of possibilities. Jessica Kingsley, London

Senior P Croall J 1993 Helping to heal: the arts in health care. Calouste Gulbenkian Foundation, London

---

CONTACT ADDRESSES

99

The Center for Health Design
PO Box 3589
Walnut Creek CA 94598-3589
USA http://healthdesign.org/

Society for the Arts in Healthcare
3867 Tennyson Street
Denver CO 80212-210, USA
http://
www.societyartshealthcare.org/

Arts for Health
Manchester Metropolitan
University
All Saints
Oxford Road
Manchester M15 6BY

13 Geopathic stress

Dawn Freshwater

Geopathic Stress – *Energies that emanate from the earth which may adversely affect general health and well-being.*

'As the eagle was killed by the arrow winged with his own feather, so the hand of the world is wounded by its own skill' Keller (1951)

INTRODUCTION

Our physical environment has changed radically with the recent evolutionary past; alongside this patterns of disease and mortality have also changed. Thanks to improvements in living conditions and enormous advances in medicine some of the great killers of days gone by have almost disappeared. In their place we are left with the diseases of civilization; one such dis-ease is that of stress (Martin 1997). Stress as a factor in ill health is now widely accepted and is well documented along with its effects on the body (Kort 1994, Ursin 1994, Martin 1997). What is not so well known is the true range of causes. This chapter discusses one of the lesser-known aspects of stress: geopathic stress. An introduction to the concept of geopathic stress is given and its influence upon ill health and the implications of this for the individual's healing process are explored. In examining this concept in more depth the philosophy of Eastern traditions will be drawn upon to incorporate the notion of the body's subtle energy system (the etheric body, chakras and meridians).

BACKGROUND

The word 'geopathic' is derived from the Greek words: *geo* (of the earth) and *pathos* (suffering or disease), hence the literal meaning of the word geopathic is suffering/disease of the earth. The term geopathic stress is generally used to describe energies that emanate from the earth which may cause ill health in human beings. The notion of earth energies is not a new one; in ancient times many Eastern cultures held the belief that there were pathways of energy, the earth's spiritual pulse, running through the landscape (Hope 1997). This belief is the basis for the science of geomancy and the ancient Chinese geomantic system *feng shui*. Interest in geopathic stress in the Western world dates back to the early 1920s.

In 1922 an English businessman, Alfred Watkins, claimed to have rediscovered an energy system that connected all the sacred centres of England. He termed this system ley lines. At approximately the same time in Germany Gustav Von Pohl discovered a link between areas with a high incidence of cancer cases and geological faults (Von Pohl 1922). Until recently, much of the research surrounding geopathic stress and its relationship to ill health has emanated from the Continent (Thurnell-Read 1994). However, the UK took a progressive stance when, in 1989, a group opposed to the building of large electric substations was formed, entitled Powerwatch UK. Today, this group coordinates a strategic nationwide approach to health hazards and has done much to attract the media's attention to the health hazards of electromagnetic fields. It is now well known that stress from electricity substations can travel down geopathic stress lines and that geopathic stress can propagate along power lines and railway tracks (National Radiological Protection Board 1992). In accounting for diseases of civilization, such as geopathic stress, some writers claim there is a mismatch between our biological makeup and the current environment (Martin 1997). It is this mismatch that will now be expanded upon in order to discover what, if any, are the implications of geopathic stress for health care professionals and the healing environment.

GEOPATHIC ENERGY

The earth has its own natural magnetic field, which is produced as the earth rotates. Electric currents are created in the molten metals found within the earth's core, as if it had a big magnet at its centre. Humans, animals and plants are accustomed to living with this magnetic field, with many mammals and animals synchronizing with the energy of the magnetic field for migration and navigation purposes. A dynamic phenomenon, the magnetic field is in a process of continuous change as it responds to changing seasons and other natural variations of the earth's rotation. Electromagnetic radiation is also a part of man's environment and includes such phenomena as sunlight, radiowaves and microwaves (Sheldrake 1988, Smith 1997).

Neither geopathic nor electromagnetic energies are visible and as yet it is difficult to quantify their effects on human beings; as a result research that has been conducted in this area has been met with much scepticism (Thurnell-Read 1995). The benefits of electromagnetic radiation for human health are well documented and enjoyed by many of us (Freshwater 1997). There is, however, an increasing body of evidence suggesting that these energies also have a detrimental effect on our health (National Radiological Protection Board 1992, Von Pohl

1993, Bachmann 1995, Thurnell-Read 1995). The human body can and does act as a receiver for electromagnetic waves; research has demonstrated that continual exposure to these waves has a deleterious effect on the natural defence mechanisms and immunity of human beings. The National Radiological Protection Board (1992) reported that those people living close to power lines were at risk of an increased incidence of headaches, depression, allergies, anxiety, irritability, fetal abnormalities and an increased risk of tumour growth or cancer. The average person is subjected to this type of electromagnetic pollution everyday in their day to day activities, for example watching TV, using microwave ovens and working on computers. Electromagnetic pollution causes the body to experience stress and renders it more vulnerable to other stresses such as geopathic stress (although Powerwatch opposition groups are currently challenging this).

Occurring as a result of natural or man made disturbances in the earth's magnetic field, for example ley lines (see Freshwater 1997), geopathic stress is thought to undermine the body's natural defences (Thurnell-Read 1995). Hence, whilst geopathic stress may not cause illness, it weakens the body providing a fertile ground in which ill health can flourish. Defences are challenged and the individual is less able to resist the insult of illnesses, viruses and bacteria (Sheldrake 1988). The body's subtle energy system and its own electrical system are affected concurrently. Furthermore, some individuals may be more at risk of ill health as a result of electromagnetic pollution, experiencing hypersensitivity (allergic) reactions to electricity (Smith 1997).

THE BODY'S OWN ENERGY SYSTEMS

Traditionally, Western science tends to view the body in physical terms, regarding it solely as a structure of flesh, blood and bones. In comparison, some traditions, especially those of the East, believe that the human has a 'subtle' body that exists alongside the physical body and has its own energy. As the physical body is permeated by nerves, so the subtle body is pervaded by thousands of channels, through which flow the winds of energy, known as *prana* (Hope 1997). The energy, which is believed to be absorbed through the acupuncture meridian lines, is known as chi and is seen as the basis of the life-force. The central channel runs from the crown of the head down to the base of the spine, along which there are seven energy wheels known as *chakras*. Acupuncture meridian lines are electromagnetic in nature and are therefore susceptible to disturbance from environmental energies. Eastern traditions give credence to the belief that the meridian lines form the interface between the physical and the ethereal, spiritual and emotional bodies, which together are termed the subtle bodies. It is the chakra system that acts as the mediator between the subtle bodies and the physical body. When the chakra system is interfered with by electromagnetic pollution and geopathic stress, essential connections between the subtle bodies may not occur, leaving the physical body weakened and prone to ill health (Gerber 1988).

On a purely physical level, geopathic stress has the potential to interfere with the body's own electrical system, including the electrical impulse that maintains the heartbeat. These sensitive electrical systems are easily influenced by external electromagnetic waves and can have an adverse effect on the body's internal magnetic mechanisms constantly striving towards homeostasis. Whilst this is of concern to us all, it has far reaching implications for the patient who is undergoing hospital treatment. Hospitalized patients are exposed to large amounts of electrical emissions and may be prone to geopathic stress. Hospitals may be located in areas of negative geopathic energy or *sha*, with particular beds positioned in high level stress zones. As hospitalized patients are usually experiencing an insult to their defence mechanisms it would be reasonable to assume that geopathic stress may impact the healing and mortality rates in certain hospitals and indeed specific departments. As an area for future research, it would be interesting to note the correlation between areas of negative earth energy and the incidence of hospital acquired infection.

THE HEALING ENVIRONMENT

Section Two of this book does much to raise awareness of the importance of the environment as a precursor to healing (see contributions by Biley (Chapter 12) and Sayre-Adams & Wright (Chapter 10)). As already mentioned, geopathic stress could be a significant factor in the consideration of hospitals as healing environments. For this reason attention is required not only to the design of hospital buildings, but also to the location of the building itself. A building constructed on negative earth energy, a term frequently referred to as 'sick building syndrome', is likely to be as sick as the patient (Moore 1992). One could also question the impact of such negative energy on the health of the staff working within such environments.

The idea that buildings may suffer from 'sickness' is a relatively recent development. Sick building syndrome, now considered a serious health risk, is thought to affect thousands of workers on a daily basis (Wilson & Hedge 1987). Interestingly, reported symptoms of sick building syndrome correlate with the symptoms of over-exposure to electromagnetic emissions (Morrow 1992, Bachmann 1995, Freshwater 1997, Biley & Freshwater 1998).

It is perhaps unrealistic to expect hospitals to relocate to areas of reduced electromagnetic pollution and geopathic stress to reduce the potential of sick building syndrome. However, it may be worth investing in some simple detective and corrective techniques in the hope that not only the patients' health might be improved, but also that the staff find themselves working in a healing environment as well as creating one.

FINDING SOLUTIONS

Many of us sense that the earth is in some way sacred and recognize the importance of living in harmony with the earth's energy. In order to create lines of positive life-enhancing energy or *sha* in healing environments, negative energy needs to first be detected. Areas of negative energy which create geopathic stress can be detected via a variety of means, including kinesiology (muscle testing), sensing (psychic responses), dowsing (using rods or pendulums) and observing animal and plant behaviour. Correcting areas of negative energy can have a positive effect on both the healing environment and on individual patients' health (Thurnell-Read 1995).

There are several simple corrective techniques that can be employed, many derived from the Chinese art of *feng shui*. The concept of chi is central to the practice of feng shui which attempts to harmonize the energy of buildings and landscapes by concentrating on enabling the free flow of chi through the environment. Chi energy can be changed through the use of mirrors, colours, gemstones and magnets (Freshwater 1997).

In siting new hospitals consideration should be given to the influence of negative earth energies, particularly in relation to the location of departments and equipment; for example, careful siting of radiographic equipment in order to minimize the impact of electromagnetic pollution on vulnerable and recuperating bodies. This is an area that Smith (1997) pays attention to in his work on the electrically sensitive patient. Smith (1997) clearly outlines the role of the nurse in caring for patients with electrical hypersensitivity, and emphasizes the need for nurses to recognize the 'triggers' within the healing environment.

Current trends indicate a drive to provide evidence of the benefits of such techniques as kinesiology, dowsing and feng shui. To date, many of the benefits are criticized as being based on anecdotal evidence. However, with the paradigm shift that is taking place in research perhaps this 'narrative' evidence could be more rigorously examined (Biley & Freshwater 1999).

Summary

This chapter has been concerned with the potential threat to the patient's well-being from geopathic stress. The concepts of geopathic stress and electromagnetic pollution present a challenge to nurses and other health care professionals in the understanding of how the physical body interacts with the environment. It has also been posited that we are more than just a physical body, we are also all that we cannot see; this includes the ethereal body, the chakras and the meridians, collectively known as the subtle bodies. This is an added dimension and one that cannot be ignored when working towards holistic healing practices with diseases, often of our own creation. Finally, there is little doubt that geopathic stress is a poorly understood phenomena and one which requires further investigation and substantive research.

REFERENCES

Bachmann M O 1995 Influences on sick building syndrome symptoms in three buildings. Social Science and Medicine 40 (2): 245–251

Biley F C Freshwater D 1999 Trends in nursing and midwifery research and the need for change in complementary therapy research. Complementary Therapies in Nursing and Midwifery 5: 99–102

Biley F C Freshwater D 1998 Spiritual care and the environment: a new paradigm for nursing? Complementary Therapies in Nursing and Midwifery 4: 98–99

Freshwater D (1997) Geopathic stress. Complementary Therapies in Nursing and Midwifery 3: 160–162

Gerber R 1988 Vibrational medicine. Bear, London

Hope J 1997 The secret language of the soul. Chronicle, San Francisco

Keller H 1951 The story of my life. Hodder and Stoughton, London

Kort W J 1994 The effect of stress on the immune response. Advanced Neuro-immunology 4: 1

Martin P 1997 The sickening mind. Brain behaviour immunity and disease, Harper Collins, London

Moore T 1992 Care of the soul. Harper Collins, New York

Morrow L A 1992 Sick building syndrome and related workplace disorders. Otolaryngology and Head and Neck Surgery 106 (6): 649–654

National Radiological Protection Board 1992 Electromagnetic fields and the risk of cancer. National Radiological Protection Board, Oxon

Sheldrake R 1988 The presence of the past: Morphic resonance and the habits of nature. Times Books, New York

Smith C W 1997 Nursing the electrically sensitive patient. Complementary Therapies in Nursing and Midwifery 3: 111–116

Thurnell-Read J 1994 Geopathic stress. International Journal of Alternative and Complementary Medicine April

Thurnell-Read J 1995 Geopathic stress. Element, Dorset

Ursin H 1994 Stress distress and immunity. Annals of New York Academic Science 741: 204

Von Pohl G 1922 Earth currents: causative factors of cancer and other diseases. French-Verlag, Stuttgart

Wilson S Hedge A 1987 The office environment survey: a study of building sickness. Building Use Studies, London

---

USEFUL ADDRESSES

Powerwatch UK
Orchard House
High Common,
Barshaw
Beccles NR34 8HW

Chartered Institution of Building
Services Engineers
Delta House
222 Balham High Road
London SW12 9BS

14 Spiritual healing research

Daniel J Benor

INTRODUCTION

The use of spiritual healing is new to modern nursing and medicine; however, it is one of the oldest known therapies, used in every culture around the world. It has been called 'faith' healing by religious groups and the media, 'paranormal' healing in Europe, 'psychic' healing in the USA, and is found in the *Index Medicus* as 'mental' healing. These and many other names testify to the lack of clarity about the mechanisms for spiritual healing. Despite our inability to explain healing, this complementary therapy has one of the largest bodies of research to support its efficacy.

Healing has been largely ignored or rejected by Western medicine because it is alien to conventional ways of relating to health and illness; however, England is a world leader in integrating healing with conventional medicine. Since the 1950s, healers have joined organizations which now have a standard Code of Conduct and, since the 1970s, healers have been allowed (by a governmental decision) to treat patients in hospitals. Their acceptance has gradually grown to the point that doctors now refer patients to healers for treatment. Some healers now work in doctors' surgeries and in hospital pain, cardiac rehabilitation and cancer centres. Only a few of these healers are paid for their work under the National Health Service.

Healing is a safe treatment, with no known deleterious effects, although there may be occasional temporary increases in pain with the first treatment or two. Healers generally view such pain as a positive sign, indicating that the body is starting to shift whatever is causing the pain, and knowing that with further treatments the pain is likely to improve. A measure of the safety of healing is the annual cost for malpractice insurance, about £6 p.a. for coverage equivalent to that of a physician, who has to pay over £1000 p.a. for the same coverage.

Healing can alleviate symptoms and help people recover from almost any illness. Regrettably, healing is often viewed as a treatment of last resort in chronic illness which has not responded to all conventional approaches. This is unfortunate because healing can be most beneficial when given early in the course of illness and is best known for its help in relieving pains from a range of causes such as tension headaches, neuralgias, arthritis, migraines and cancers. The swelling and physical disabilities of rheumatoid and osteoarthritis, for instance, also respond well to healing. Anxiety is also a symptom which responds well to healing.

PROCESS OF HEALING

Spiritual healing is generally given in one of two ways:

    laying-on of hands
    distant healing.

In laying-on of hands, healers may hold their hands near to but not touching the body, or only lightly touching the body. They quiet their minds and focus mentally on being available to help and heal the patient. When undergoing a treatment of healing, most healers report that patients flush, sigh and relax within minutes of the commencement of treatment.

In distant ('absent' or non-local) healings, healers send healing mentally – as meditation, prayer, or healing wishes – from a location which can be many miles away from the patient.

The media have focused largely on 'miraculous' cures, where changes in chronic and serious illnesses have occurred very rapidly. The more usual course is for changes to occur gradually, with treatments given weekly over several months.

APPROACHES TO HEALING

Therapeutic touch

There are many varieties of healing available. One of the most familiar is therapeutic touch (TT), developed by Dolores Krieger, a nurse based at New York University, together with Dora Kunz, a gifted, intuitive healer. Tens of thousands of nurses and other carers have learned to administer TT healing and Certification is now available to TT practitioners and well established in the UK (Sayre-Adams & Wright 1995) The largest number of research studies in humans has been done with TT (see also chapter 33, Therapeutic Touch).

Reiki

Reiki, derived from Japanese traditions, is another popular healing method. Reiki is taught by Masters. Originally, Reiki Masters were carefully chosen, but today it would seem that nearly anyone can become a Master by taking a brief course, and the selection is often not very rigorous, which may give cause for concern.

Shamanism

Shamanism has been practised for many thousands of years in every part of the world. It is rich in healing lore, and may include chanting, dancing and many other practices. Without research, it is difficult to know whether elements of shamanic healings are effective interventions or simply culturally defined placebos (see also Chapter 11, Shamanism).

BRITISH ORGANIZATIONS

In the UK there are many healing groups within the Confederation of Healing Organisations. The largest is the National Federation of Spiritual Healers (NFSH), numbering over 5000 members. The NFSH trains and certifies its healers, teaching trainees clinical approaches and the Code of Conduct, and supervising the development of their healing gifts in healing centres around the country.

THE NEED FOR HEALING RESEARCH

As with any treatment modality, be it medical, surgical, or social, it is not possible to know whether it is effective without formal studies. The power of suggestion alone can frequently produce dramatic self-healing effects in many illnesses (Benor 1993, 2000). Controlled studies, in which a treatment is compared with no treatment or with a treatment of established value, confirm the efficacy of a treatment.

Conventional medicine is sceptical about treatments that are not taught in medical and nursing schools. Indeed the author, trained in psychology, medicine, psychiatry and research, was very sceptical of healing prior to a detailed review of the controlled studies that confirmed healing effects. In addition to the controlled studies, there are qualitative studies exploring the perceived experiences of healers and of recipients of healing.

Research examples

The author identified 197 controlled studies of healing, showing significant effects in humans, animals, plants, bacteria, yeasts, cells in laboratory culture, enzymes and DNA (Benor 1992, 2000).

Here are a few examples of studies of healing in humans:

Study 1

Following a pilot study, Michael Dixon, a GP in Devon, recruited 57 patients in his surgery. All had chronic conditions (at least 6 months), including arthritis, neck/back pain, depression, psoriasis, migraine/head pain, stress and other problems. A research nurse assigned patients alternately to treatment and control groups after obtaining their consent to participate. Out of 73 patients referred by their GP to the study, 30 treatment and 27 control group patients were entered in the study. Treatment groups were similar in duration and severity of problems.

An NFSH healer gave 40 minutes of healing weekly for 10 weeks. She discussed each patient's symptoms and general well-being, then gave healing with her hands passing several inches over the body while she visualized white light passing through her to the patient. The control group patients received routine care from their doctor, and were given healing 12 or 24 weeks later.

All patients were assessed at the start of the study and at 3 months on the Hospital Anxiety and Depression (HAD) scale (Zigmond/Snaith), and for physical and mental function on the Nottingham Health Profile (S Hunt). At 6 months all the treatment and half the control group patients were assessed again. In addition, patients scored their symptoms with the research nurse on a scale of 0 (no symptoms) to 10 (unbearable), and were asked to report any changes they perceived in their symptoms at 3 and 6 months. Immune functions were assessed by assays of natural killer cells (CD16 and CD56).[1] The numbers of medical visits for both groups of patients in the year prior to starting the study were compared with those during the 6 months following the study. The research staff was not blind to treatment and control conditions.

Results After receiving healing for 3 months, the treatment group scored significantly better on symptoms scores ($P < 0.01$–0.05). No significant differences were found at 6 months between the treatment and control groups. The self-assessments of 'whether they thought their symptoms had improved or deteriorated' showed significantly more improvements in the treatment group compared to the control group at 3 months ($P < 0.01$) and at 6 months ($P < 0.05$).

Treatment group affective states improved significantly more than controls for both anxiety ($P < 0.01$)[2] and depression ($P < 0.05$)[3] scales at 3 months, and at 6 months for both anxiety ($P < 0.01$)[4] and depression ($P < 0.05$) scales.[5]

---

[1] At the half-way point in the study it was discovered that the chemicals for measuring CD16 were faulty. It took several months to sort this out, and therefore the healing for the C patients in the second half of the study was delayed to 6 months rather than 3 months, allowing comparison with E patients just after they finished their treatments, as well as 3 months later.
[2] Median score, treatment group: 4.0, IQR 1.0 to 5.0; control group 0, IQR −2.0 to 2.0, Treatment difference: 3.0, CI 2.0, 5.0; T = 523.5.
[3] Median score, Treatment group: 2.0, IQR 0 to 4.0; control group 0 to 1.0, Treatment difference: 2.0, CI 0 to 3.0, T = 445.0.
[4] Treatment difference: 3.0, CI 0 to 4.0, T = 226.5.
[5] Treatment difference: 2.0, CI 0 to 4.0, T = 207.0.

The percentages of CD56 and CD16 cells did not significantly change during the study for treated or control groups.

In summarizing the study, Dixon (1998) observed that 52% of patients reported substantial improvements after healing, when they had previously been unresponsive to conventional treatments. None were worse. After 6 months the general sense of well-being was better maintained than the improvements in specific symptoms.

This pilot study attracted a lot of attention in the media because Dixon also noted that over a 6-month period in the pilot study, healing treatments for 25 patients saved the surgery over £1000 in medication costs.

Study 2

Keller & Bzdek (1986) studied the effects of TT on tension headache pain.

The patients were 60 volunteers between the ages of 18 and 59 (mean 30). To be included they had to have tension headache, 'defined as dull, persistent head pain, usually bilateral, with feelings of heaviness, pressure, or tightness, which did not involve a prodrome, neurologic deficit, infectious process, or recent head trauma' and had to be free of headache medication during the 4 hours preceding the study. Patients were randomly assigned to TT or placebo touch groups and were blind regarding their treatments. Subjective experience of headache pain was evaluated on three scales of the McGill-Melzack Pain Questionnaire (MMPQ). The MMPQ was completed just prior to and 5 minutes after the treatments.

For the TT group, the researcher centred herself and passed her hands 6–12 inches away from the subjects without touching them, 'to assess the energy field which extends beyond the skin and to redirect areas of accumulated tension out of the field. She then let her hands rest around, but not on, the head or solar plexus in areas of energy imbalance or deficit and directed life energy to the subject.' For the mock TT (MTT) group the researcher simulated the above procedure, omitting the therapeutic components, focusing her mind on subtraction of 7s from 100, while holding no intent to help in her consciousness. Subjects in both groups sat quietly and were asked to breathe slowly during the 5-minute procedures.

The initial severity of headaches was comparable between the two groups, which showed a difference of no more than a half-point on the three scales of the MMPQ. Significant results were found in 28 (90%) patients, who had reduced headache pain on post-test compared to pre-test scores on all three MMPQ tests, both 5 minutes and 4 hours after TT treatments ($P < 0.0001$).[6]

---

[6]Wilcoxon signed rank test for differences.

Significant effects were also shown on all three MMPQ tests ($P < 0.005$ on PRI scale ($P < 0.002$ on NWC; and $P < 0.0001$ on PPI test) comparing the TT group with MTT group immediately after treatments.[7] The superiority of TT over MTT at 4 hours after interventions was not supported on the initial data analysis. However, researchers found that the placebo group had 15 subjects (50%) who 'used treatments [unspecified] to relieve their headache during the 4-hour interval between post-test and delayed post-test, but only five subjects (16%) in the TT group reported an intervening treatment.' Removing data of all who used other treatments from the analysis, significant differences between the groups became apparent ($P < 0.005$–0.01) depending on the particular MMPQ test.

Correlations of patients' responses were sought with age, sex, practice of meditation, religion and level of initial scepticism toward TT. With one exception on one test, no correlations were found.[8]

Subjects in the TT group reported sensations of tingling, warmth and relaxation, though they had not been told what to expect and had no prior experience with TT. Subjects in the placebo group reported a lesser reduction of pain and more often used other treatments. 'Thus it appears that although the placebo intervention did reduce headache pain, the effect did not occur as often, was not as great and did not last as long as the effect of TT' (Keller & Bzdek 1986).

Some of the best human studies confirm the effects of distant healing:

Sicher et al (1998) demonstrated in a double-blind, randomized study of distant healing that patients with AIDS who received healing had significantly fewer AIDS-related illnesses ($P < 0.04$) and lower severity of illnesses ($P < 0.02$). Visits to doctors were significantly less frequent ($P < 0.01$), as were hospitalizations ($P < 0.04$) and days in hospital ($P < 0.04$). Mood was assessed on the Profile of Mood States (POMS). Again there was significantly more improvement in the healing group ($P < 0.02$). Improvements were noted on four out of six subscales, including depression, tension, confusion and fatigue. A higher mean score (not significant) was found in the treatment group at baseline. This could have contributed to the greater improvement shown in mood.[9]

This excellent study confirms that healing can be effective when projected from a distance. Hopefully, people with AIDS will be able to have the benefits of spiritual healing.

[7]Wilcoxon rank sum test.
[8]'The one exception was the post-test difference on the PPI scale in the placebo group, which was inversely correlated with years of education, $r = -0.53$, $P < 0.002$.'
[9]CD4 immune cell counts and scores on the Wahler Physical Symptom Inventory (PPSI), and a Medical Outcomes Survey (MOS) for AIDS measured quality of life did not differ significantly between the two groups.

Test your own healing abilities

- Plant seeds from the same source
- Use three pots with soil from the same source, taking care to place seeds with pointy ends down, at the same depth in all pots
- Water each with the same amount of water, keeping them under identical light sources
- Send healing wishes to the first pot, leave the second alone
- Send negative thoughts to the third
- After 2 weeks you may see marked differences between the amount

Healing research in nursing

It is not surprising that the primary practitioners of TT healing in the USA are nurses, with TT healing being taught at 90 schools of nursing. The popularity of TT is not due only to the fact that one of its originators, Dolores Krieger, was a nurse but also because TT provides nurses with a tool to alleviate pain, anxiety and other symptoms, and to facilitate recovery from many illnesses. A large body of the available research has been done by nurses, mostly as master's theses and doctoral dissertations. Among these are studies of healing for pain, anxiety (in adults, children, and neonates), milk letdown in nursing mothers, and more (See Benor 2000, and chapter 21, Healing, this book).

Nurses have also been pioneers in exploring the perceived experience of healing through qualitative research (Barrington 1985, Heidt 1990, Samarel 1992).

CONCLUSION

Healing is safe as well as effective. There are no known deleterious effects of healing. Witness to this is the low cost of malpractice insurance for healers in the UK (under £10 p.a.).

Healing has been found effective for treatment of:

- headaches
- backaches
- postoperative pain (Wirth et al 1993a)
- arthritis (functional disabilities as well as pain)
- wound healing (Wirth et al 1993b)
- anxiety (Gulak 1985)
- bereavement (Quinn 1993).

Summary

In the UK, the Confederation of Healing Organisations and major healing organizations in the country, has a Code of Conduct for its members which has been recognized by the Royal Colleges of Physicians, Surgeons, Nurses and Midwifery. Many of the healing organizations teach healing, as does the Didsbury Trust (see chapter 33, Therapeutic Touch). Healers can provide treatment which is complementary to conventional medical care. Healing is a safe and effective treatment which will hopefully find increasing use as a complement to conventional medical care.

REFERENCES

Barrington M R 1985 A slip in time and place. Fate (Oct): 88–94

Benor D J 1992 Healing research, Vol. I. Helix Books, Munich

Benor D J 1993 Healing research, Vol. II. Helix Books, Munich

Benor D J 2000 Healing research, Vols. I–II (revised edn). Vision Publications, Southfield, MI

Dixon M 1998 Does 'healing' benefit patients with chronic symptoms? A quasi-randomized trial in general practice. Journal of the Royal Society of Medicine 91: 183–188

Gulak J 1985 Lowering the anxiety levels in persons undergoing bioergotherapy. Psychotronika 6–9 (translated from Polish by Alexander Imich)

Heidt P R 1990 Openness: a qualitative analysis of nurses' and patients' experiences of therapeutic touch. Image: Journal of Nursing Scholarship 22 (3): 180–186

Keller E Bzdek V M 1986 Effects of therapeutic touch on tension headache pain. Nursing Research 35: 101–104

Quinn J F 1993 Psychoimmunologic effects of therapeutic touch on practitioners and recently bereaved recipients: a pilot study. Advances in Nursing Science 15: 13–26

Sayre-Adams J Wright S 1995 The theory and practice of therapeutic touch. Churchill Livingstone, Edinburgh

Samarel N 1992 The experience of receiving therapeutic touch. Journal of Advanced Nursing 17: 651–657

Sicher F Targ E Moore D et al 1998 A randomized, double-blind study of the effects of distant healing in a population with advanced AIDS. Western Journal of Medicine 169 (6): 356–363

Wirth D P Brenlan D R Levine R J Rodriguez C M 1993a The effect of complementary healing therapy on postoperative pain after surgical removal of impaqcted third molar teeth. Complementary Therapies in Medicine 1: 133–138

Wirth D P Richardson J T Eidelman W C O'Malley A C 1993b Full-thickness dermal wounds treated with non-contact therapeutic touch: a replication and extension. Complementary Therapies in Medicine 1: 127–132

USEFUL ADDRESSES

National Federation of Spiritual
Healers
Old Manor Farm Studio
Church Street
Sunbury-on-Thames
Middlesex TW16 6RG
Tel: 01932 783164
E-mail: office@nfsh.org.uk

Confederation of Healing
Organisations
The Red and White House
113 High Street
Berkhampstead
Hertfordshire HP4 2DJ
Tel: 01442 870660

SECTION 3

Therapies

15 Acupuncture

Stephanie Downey

Acupuncture – *a Chinese medical system which aims to diagnose illness and promote health by stimulating the body's self-healing powers.*

In the last three decades there has been a significant increase in the acceptance of acupuncture within Western medical practice. Recognized by the British Medical Association (BMA) as a 'discrete clinical discipline' (BMA 1993), acupuncture now faces the challenge of biomedical integration and the need to adapt to Western needs whilst still retaining the integrity of its oriental tradition.

Acupuncture involves the insertion of fine needles into specific points on the body. The word derives from the Latin *acus* (needle) and *punctura* (puncture). Behind this apparently simple technique, lies a rich and complex theoretical system rooted in Confucian and Taoist philosophy and developed and refined over 2000 years through extensive observation and clinical evaluation.

Central to the theory behind acupuncture is the concept of the body as a self-healing, self-rectifying, dynamic whole, a network of interrelating and interacting energies (Firebrace & Hill 1988). The even distribution and flow of these energies maintains health, and through the insertion of needles acupuncture helps the body to correct itself by realigning or redirecting the energy. A related technique, moxibustion, involves the application of heat from the burning of the herb mugwort (*Artemisia vulgaris*) at the acupuncture points. This has a warming, moving and strengthening effect on the body.

Acupuncture is but one aspect of traditional Chinese medicine that includes herbs, diet, massage and exercise. All of these techniques developed on the basis of principles which see the body as inseparable from its environment, a microcosm of the universe and permeated with the same energy (Beijing College of Traditional Medicine et al 1980). In the human body this energy, or Qi, is dispersed through 12 main channels (meridians) all following fixed pathways to connect the different levels from the internal organs to the skin. Illness occurs primarily when there is excess, deficiency or obstruction of the energy within the organs or meridian pathways. For example, symptoms such as arthritic pain in the hips, intercostal neuralgia or migraine headaches would suggest an imbalance in the Gall Bladder, whose meridian traverses the lateral sides of the body from the foot to the temples. Likewise, pain and stiffness in the arm of someone with repetitive strain injury may be due to blocked Qi in the Large Intestine meridian which runs from the index finger to the elbow. Similarly, a deficiency of energy in the Lungs can manifest as dyspnoea, asthma or a tendency to catch colds. The aim of acupuncture in each case is to regulate and correct imbalances of Qi and so assist the body's own recuperative powers.

The dynamic balance of energy central to acupuncture can be expressed by the concepts of Yin and Yang. In Chinese medicine, Yin/Yang describe patterns of disharmony and are relative rather than absolute terms. Yang is characterized by heat, movement, activity and excess, whereas Yin relates more to cold, sluggishness, inactivity and deficiency. A balance of each kind of energy is necessary for health.

A further refinement of Yin/Yang is the Five Elements or Phases. This is a system of correspondences which include organs/meridians, emotions, seasons and climates, linked to the elements of Fire, Earth, Metal, Water and Wood in a dynamic cycle of creation and control. For example:

- Fire: Heart/Small Intestine, joy, summer, heat
- Earth: Spleen/Stomach, obsession, late summer/between seasons, dampness
- Metal: Lungs/Large Intestine, sadness/grief, autumn, dryness
- Water: Kidney/Bladder, fear/fright, winter, cold
- Wood: Liver/Gall Bladder, anger, spring, wind.

The inter-relating energies are governed by this relationship, so that an imbalance in one area will lead to a breakdown of the cycle causing disharmony within other elements and manifesting as physical or emotional disorders within the associated organ/meridian.

The existence of Qi and channels cannot be explained, as yet, within the parameters of Western science. Acupuncture has been shown to have an effect on biochemical, neurological and hormonal systems. However, none of these paradigms is adequate to account for the permanent changes acupuncture can mobilize in some aspects of physiological behaviour; for example, in chronic headaches (Bensoussan 1991).

The World Health Organization (Bannerman 1979) recognizes the efficacy of acupuncture in the treatment of over 40 diseases. While its use in the West is often limited to chronic conditions, the integration of traditional and modern medicine in China has shown acupuncture to be remarkably successful in the treatment of more serious and acute diseases such as appendicitis, cholecystitis, renal colic and the sequelae of cerebrovascular accident (Deadman 1982, Hopwood 1996). For acupuncture to find its true place within the medical services it is important that it is used in the hospital system alongside biomedicine.

To ensure its future as a complete medical system, acupuncture faces three major issues: training, regulatory procedures and research. The British Acupuncture Council was formed in 1995, through a merger of five previous associations, to represent and govern its professionally qualified members. Common standards are set in education, ethics, discipline, and health and safety in order to ensure that the interests of the public are met at all times. The British Acupuncture Accreditation Board (BAAB) has also been established, which seeks to accredit colleges on the basis of compliance with established minimum standards of training (Shifrin 1993, Uddin 1993).

While research into acupuncture is prolific in China and has increased in the West (Bensoussan 1991), this has largely been modelled on the empirical methods that dominate the natural sciences. The extent to which Chinese medicine can be understood or evaluated within the current framework of conventional Western science requires urgent attention (Scheid 1993).

HISTORICAL BACKGROUND

The origin of acupuncture in China is not clear. Although excavations have revealed the existence of stone needles dating back to 3000 BC, the earliest document, the *Huangdi NeiJing*, was probably written between 300 and 100 BC (Maciocia 1982). Translated as the *Yellow Emperor's Classic of Internal Medicine*, this work lays down the theoretical foundations of Chinese medicine and is still frequently cited in modern acupuncture textbooks. In the second century BC acupuncture was adopted as the dominant therapeutic technique (Unschuld 1985) and later centuries saw the development of the main acupuncture theories relating to meridian systems, Yin/Yang, the Five Elements, the nature and types of Qi, the functions of the organs and their pathology. The popularity and acceptance of different schools of thought regarding Chinese medical theories varied throughout Chinese history in response to shifts in religious behaviour and sociopolitical ideologies.

After the Opium War in 1840, biomedicine as part of Western science and technology came to China and traditional medicine was marginalized. Since the formation of the People's Republic in 1949, Chinese medicine has been actively encouraged and systematized.

Knowledge of acupuncture in Europe was generally derived from reports by travelling doctors and treatises by Jesuit missionaries working in China in the seventeenth century (Hsu 1989). Gaining popularity initially in France and Germany, acupuncture spread to Britain and has become increasingly widespread since the 1960s.

TREATMENT

Although acupuncture has gained prominence in the West as a method of pain relief, its efficacy extends to disorders of the respiratory, digestive and nervous systems as well as emotional and psychological problems.

The diagnostic process, whereby signs and symptoms are pieced together and synthesized until a picture of the whole person appears, is integral to the application of acupuncture. An initial consultation will address the current problem as well as eliciting information about emotional state, exposure to adverse climatic conditions, trauma, accidents, hereditary factors, diet and social factors, all of which are seen to interact to disrupt the flow of Qi. Diagnosis will also be based on the person's appearance, facial colour and posture. Finally, the pulse will be palpated and the tongue observed to provide additional information about the energetic balance and state of Qi within the organs and meridians.

The diagnosis is made according to the theoretical framework of traditional Chinese medicine. Most important is the recognition of the

Therapeutic potential in nursing

There are many opportunities for nurses to practise acupuncture, although only a full training in traditional Chinese medicine will prevent acupuncture becoming just another biomedical technique. The nursing role may also need to be re-examined as well as the extent to which holistic care can be provided within the constraints of traditional nursing models (Burke 1993).

Potential areas for acupuncture in nursing include:

- Pain management – post-operatively, in out-patient clinics, accident and emergency departments
- Sports medicine – in conjunction with physiotherapy
- Obstetrics – pain relief, induction of labour, turning the fetus in breech presentation
- Oncology – control of emesis after chemotherapy
- Occupational health
- Mental health – emotional distress
- Drug rehabilitation centres – control of withdrawal symptoms
- Treatment of HIV/AIDS as part of a multidisciplinary team.

uniqueness of each individual's condition. Two people may present with the diagnostic label of arthritis, yet one may experience a fixed biting pain aggravated by cold and have a pale tongue and slow pulse, while the other may have migratory pain, red hot swollen joints, red tongue and a rapid pulse. The diagnosis and treatment will be tailored to the individual. As well as inserting fine needles into specific points on the body, moxibustion may be applied, and each subsequent treatment will vary in the points used, according to the particular recovery pattern. The therapeutic basis in traditional terms of acupuncture stimulation is that by restoring the flow of Qi within the channels, the 'vital energy' of the organism is regulated (reinforced or reduced) and thus restores balance, improves body resistance and helps to eliminate pathogenic factors (Hillier & Jewell 1983).

Contraindications for use

Certain behaviour is thought to affect the state of Qi and may counteract the effect of acupuncture or occasionally result in dizziness. In general the following should be avoided immediately before and directly after treatment (Luwen 1990):

- alcohol
- excessive fatigue and hunger
- large meals
- sexual activity
- hot baths
- extreme emotional states.

In pregnancy there are no absolute contraindications, but some restrictions (Zharkin 1990) as follows:

- Moxibustion is not recommended, apart from certain specific points
- Certain points should not be needled during the first and second trimesters, or points below the umbilicus on the anterior abdominal

Summary

Acupuncture has been shown to be effective in the treatment of a wide range of diseases. It may be used in a number of health care settings such as pain clinics, paediatrics and midwifery. However, care should be taken to ensure practitioners are well qualified, and where possible, acupuncture should be used to treat the whole person rather than for symptomatic relief.

REFERENCES

Bannerman R H 1979 Acupuncture: the WHO view. World Health (December): 24–29

Beijing College of Traditional Chinese Medicine et al 1980 Essentials of Chinese acupuncture. Foreign Language Press, Beijing

Bensoussan A 1991 The vital meridian. Churchill Livingstone, Melbourne

BMA 1993 Complementary medicine. Oxford University Press, Oxford

Burke C 1993 Cancer nursing: complementary/conventional approaches combine. Complementary Therapies in Medicine 1: 158–163

Deadman P 1982 Report on the first international course for further students in acupuncture and moxibustion. Journal of Chinese Medicine 9: 1–5

Firebrace P Hill S 1988 New ways to health – a guide to acupuncture. Hamlyn, London

Hillier S M Jewell J A 1983 Health care and traditional medicine in China, 1800–1982. Routledge & Kegan Paul, London, p 251

Hopwood V 1996 Acupuncture in stroke recovery: a literature review. Complementary Therapies in Medicine 4: 258–263

Hsu E 1989 Outline of the history of acupuncture in Europe. Journal of Chinese Medicine 29: 28–32

Luwen G 1990 Understanding the theory of acupuncture contraindications according to the NeiJing. Journal of Chinese Medicine 34: 31–32

Maciocia G 1982 History of acupuncture. Journal of Chinese Medicine 9: 9–15

Scheid V 1993 Orientalism revisited. European Journal of Oriental Medicine 1: 22–31

Shifrin K 1993 Setting standards for acupuncture training – a model for complementary medicine. Complementary Therapies in Medicine 1: 91–95

Uddin J 1993 The BMA report. European Journal of Oriental Medicine 1: 50–51

Unchuld P 1985 Medicine in China: a history of ideas. University of California Press, Berkeley

Zharkin N 1990 Acupuncture in obstetrics. Journal of Chinese Medicine 33: 10–13

FURTHER READING – JOURNALS

Cardini F Huang W 1998 Moxibustion for correction of breech presentation: a randomised clinical trial. Journal of the American Medical Association 280 (18): 1580–1584

Christensen P A 1989 Electro-acupuncture and post-operative pain. British Journal of Anaesthesia 62: 258–262

Huang X 1994 The treatment of 114 cases of chemotherapeutic leucopenia by cone moxibustion. Journal of Chinese Medicine 44: 22–23

Knapman J 1993 Controlling emesis after chemotherapy. Nursing Standard 7: 38–39

Lipton D S Brewington V Smith M 1994 Acupuncture for crack-cocaine detoxification: experimental evaluation of efficacy. Journal of Substance Abuse Treatment 11 (3): 205–215

Richardson P H Vincent C A 1986 Acupuncture for the treatment of pain: a review of evaluative research. Pain 24: 15–40

Schlager A Offer T Baldissera I 1998 Laser stimulation of acupuncture point P6 reduces post-operative vomiting in children undergoing strabismus surgery. British Journal of Anaesthesia 81 (4): 529–532

Taylor B 1990 Acupuncture – a balancing act. Openmind 43: 12–14

Ternov K Nilsson M Lofberg L Algotsson L Akeson J 1998 Acupuncture for pain relief during childbirth. Acupuncture and Electro Therapeutics Research 23: 19–26

Tsuei J J et al 1974 Induction of labour by acupuncture and electrical stimulation. Obstetrics and Gynaecology 43: 337–342

Woodier N C Price P 1984 Acupuncture and its role in occupational health. Occupational Health (September): 406–416

For a recent review of acupuncture research, contact the Acupuncture Research Resource Centre (details below). In conjunction with the British Acupuncture Council, ARRC has published a series of briefing papers: 'Acupuncture – the evidence for effectiveness' 1998–1999.

So far these cover acupuncture in the treatment of migraine, stroke, arthritis, gynaecology & menopause, citing clinical trials, outcome studies and case studies. The papers seek to present, discuss and critically evaluate the evidence.

FURTHER READING – BOOKS

Auteroche B et al 1992 Acupuncture and moxibustion: a guide to clinical practice. Churchill Livingstone, Edinburgh

Bensoussan A 1991 The vital meridian: a modern exploration of acupuncture. Churchill Livingstone, Melbourne

Kaptchuk T 1983 The web that has no weaver. Congdon & Weed, New York

Maciocia G 1989 The foundations of Chinese medicine. Churchill Livingstone, Edinburgh

MacPherson H Kaptchuk T (eds) 1997 Acupuncture in Practice. Case history insights from the West. Churchill Livingstone, Edinburgh

Shanghai College of Traditional Medicine 1981 Acupuncture: a comprehensive text. Eastland Press, Chicago

Trevelyan J Booth B 1994 Complementary medicine for nurses, midwives and health visitors. Macmillan Press, Houndmills, Basingstoke

USEFUL ADDRESSES

British Acupuncture Council
63 Jeddo Road
London W12 9HQ
Tel: 020 8735 0400
Fax: 020 8735 0404
E-mail: info@acupuncture.org.uk
website: www.acupuncture.org.uk

ARRC (Acupuncture Research Resource Centre)
Centre for Complementary Health Studies
University of Exeter
Amory Building
Exeter EX4 4RJ
Tel: 01392 264459
Fax: 01392 433828
E-mail: ARRC@ex.ac.uk

Accredited colleges

The College of Traditional
Acupuncture (UK)
Tao House
Queensway
Royal Leamington Spa
Warwickshire CV31 3L2
Tel: 01926 422121
Fax: 01926 888282

The International College of
Oriental Medicine UK
Green Hedges House
Green Hedges Avenue
East Grinstead West Sussex
RH19 1DZ
Tel: 01342 313106

Traditional Chinese
Medicine/Acupuncture
Centre for Community Care and
Primary Health
University of Westminster, 309
Regent Street
London W1R 8AL
Tel: 020 7911 5082

Northern College of Acupuncture
124 Acomb Road
York YO2 4EY
Tel: 01904 785120

The College of Integrated Chinese
Medicine
19 Castle Street
Reading RG1 7SB
Tel: 0118 950 8880
Fax: 0118 950 8890

The London College of Traditional
Acupuncture
HR House
447 High Road Finchley
London N12 0AF
Tel: 020 8371 0820

16 Aromatherapy

Caroline Stevensen

Aromatherapy – *Treatments using essential oils extracted from plants for therapeutic effect.*

Aromatherapy, the use of plant essential oils for health and well-being, is now a concept familiar to many nurses. Essential oils can be used to calm, uplift and heal through a variety of means including diffusion through the air, inhalation, absorption through the skin via massage (Jäger et al 1992), in a compress, mouth-rinse or used in wound care. The internal or oral use of essential oils remains the application of choice for the medical profession in France, but this is yet to come into practice in nursing care in the UK. Training, safety and prescribing issues are some of the reasons for this at present. Oral prescribing and the ingestion of oils by mouth, vagina or rectum is not current nursing practice in the UK.

There are many therapeutic essential oils. They can be used to relax or invigorate the individual, and also for specific conditions; for example:

- lavender (*Lavandula latifolia*) for first-aid of burns (Franchomme & Pénoël 1990)
- neroli (*Citrus aurantium* ssp. *aurantium*) for anxiety (Franchomme & Pénoël 1990, Stevensen 1994)
- tea tree (*Maleleuca alternifolia*) for its antibacterial and antifungal action (Franchomme & Pénoël 1990).

How essential oils work is not entirely understood at present despite scientific research, but this does not necessarily detract from their therapeutic value (Valnet 1990). It is thought that chemical properties of the essential oils, when absorbed in the body, have certain therapeutic benefits. Some therapists believe that the essential oil is the 'soul' of the plant, having both powerful and subtle properties that uplift the spirit as well as assisting with more fundamental health problems of body and mind.

HISTORICAL BACKGROUND

The use of plant extracts for health and well-being has been documented since records began. It is estimated that as far back as 40 000 years, Australian aborigines developed a knowledge of native plants for medicinal purposes which is still in use today. An example is the valuable antibacterial and antifungal properties of the Australian tea tree (*Maleleuca alternifolia terpineol-4*), the essential oil of which is used in modern aromatherapy (Blackwell 1991, Franchomme & Pénoël 1990). Many ancient civilizations have used aromatic products. In 4500 BC, Kiwant Ti, a Chinese emperor, recorded therapeutic properties of plants that match those ascribed to them today (Arcier 1990). The ancient Egyptians used herbal oils to embalm bodies in preparation for the next life. Priests of that period were also doctors and used herbs and oils for the treatment of the sick as well as for beauty (Tisserand 1980). In the Bible, many references are made to plant oils. Moses was instructed to make a holy anointing oil from myrrh, calamus, cinnamon, cassia and olive oil (Exodus: chapter 30, verses 22–26). Frankincense and myrrh were reported to have been brought to the Christ child at his birth (Gospel according to St Matthew: chapter 2, verse 11). Plant oils continued to be used down the ages by the Hebrews, Greeks and Romans. Hippocrates, the father of modern medicine, several hundred years BC, commended a daily scented bath and massage for good health.

The first distillation of essential oils is formally attributed to the Arab scholar, Avicenna, in the tenth century AD. However, archeological evidence from the Indus Valley civilization suggests that this technique was known 5000 years earlier (Williams 1989). The use of plant oils continued throughout the Middle Ages up to modern times. Therapeutic use of essential oils this century is attributed to the French chemist R M Gattefosse (Franchomme & Pénoël 1990). After severely burning his hand in a laboratory accident, he plunged it into a vat of lavender oil to find that the wound healed remarkably quickly and with no scarring. He coined the term 'aromathérapie' and his book of the same name describing his discoveries and experiences was published in 1931. Further research was carried out by Dr Jean Valnet in the 1960s, and the publication of his book *The practice of aromatherapy* (Valnet 1990) began a new wave of interest in the subject. The use of aromatherapy in nursing was a developing trend through the 1980s. The increasing amount of nursing research on the clinical effectiveness of aromatherapy is encouraging (Dunn 1992, Buckle 1993, Dale & Cornwall 1994, Stevensen 1994, Corner et al 1995, Evans 1995, Wilkinson 1995, Hudson 1996), although more clinical trials are needed.

TREATMENT

The properties of essential oils

The chemical properties of essential oils have been categorized by Franchomme & Pénoël (1990) according to the functional group theory. In this system, the following therapeutic properties have been attributed to the chemical components of the oils:

- Alcohols (C10): nervous system tonics, anti-infectious+++, immunostimulants
- Alcohols (C15–C20): oestrogen-like action
- Aldehydes: sedatives, anti-infectious, litholytic
- Aromatic aldehydes: anti-infectious+++, immunostimulants
- Coumarins and lactones: sedative, calming and anticoagulant
- Esters: relaxants, antispasmodics
- Ketones: mucolytic, lipolytic and cicatrizing
- Oxides: expectorants, antiparasitic
- Phenols: balance the autonomic nervous system, antispasmodics, anti-infectious+++, immunostimulants
- Terpenes (C10): cortisone-like action
- Terpenes (C15): antihistamine, antiallergic.

Currently there is some dispute regarding the accuracy of these associations. Indeed Tisserand (1998/9) has challenged the current scientific aromatherapists to give good evidence for what is known as the functional group theory of essential oil chemical constituents. Some of these chemicals, such as ketones and phenols, can be toxic in large quantities or in patients with certain conditions, for example pregnancy or epilepsy. Understanding the chemical components of each oil is a necessary part of professional aromatherapy. For example, rosemary (*Rosmarinus officinalis*) essential oil has differing levels of toxicity depending on its chemotype or chemical subgrouping; the verbenone form has a higher risk of ketone toxicity than the borneone form.

The entire issue of the safety of essential oils has been discussed in detail by Tisserand & Balacs (1995), but statements in this text are now being challenged by Guba (1998) who claims that aromatherapists have become overcautious with respect to the actual dangers of essential oils. This debate will no doubt go on well into the new millennium until enough research has been done to satisfy all parties.

The quality and chemical contents of essential oils are determined by their conditions, altitude and weather patterns during growth, as well as the method of extraction. Essential oils are extracted principally by distillation, but other methods such as maceration, expression and solvent extraction are used depending on the source of the oil. Essential oils should be grown organically without chemical fertilizers and distilled without the addition of any other chemicals. Essential oils can be adulterated or extended with synthetic chemicals to increase productivity or to stabilize the perfume (as is required in the cosmetic industry). This will reduce or remove therapeutic effect and increase levels of toxicity in some oils. In addition, if the process of distillation is cut short, some therapeutic effects may be lost as more time is needed to extract certain chemical components. For example, if distillation is incomplete some of the sedating and calming effects of lactones and coumarins contained in lavender oil may be lost.

Information in the form of safety data sheets about the source of essential oils and standard of production should be available from any company selling them for therapeutic purposes. Poorly produced and identified oils could place patients at risk of skin reactions or more serious toxic reactions. Each essential oil has internationally accepted levels for its chemical components, which can be analysed by liquid gas chromatography (Williams 1989, Franchomme & Pénoël 1990). It should be possible to obtain all this information from a reliable supplier.

So concerned about the safety of essential oils are some hospitals and health authorities in the UK, that some nurses (Fowler & Wall 1997, 1998) have adopted the use of safety risk assessments usually used in hospitals for hazardous substances. These regulations are known as Control of Substances Hazardous to Health (COSHH) and the Chemical Hazard Information and Packaging for Supply (CHIPS). In their discussion, the authors conclude that the chemical risks of essential oils are probably less significant than those associated with other practices and that these should not be taken out of proportion; however, some risk may be present.

STORAGE OF ESSENTIAL OILS

Essential oils must be stored in amber glass bottles as their constituents are affected by light. Blue glass tones, whilst attractive, do not cut out damaging rays from light that would affect the oils adversely. Plastic containers can adversely affect oils. As essential oils are volatile and evaporate easily, bottles should be firmly sealed and stored away from heat. Undiluted oils will keep for several years, whilst diluted oils may keep up to 12 months if stored correctly.

Administration of essential oils

There are several methods by which aromatherapy can be administered in a nursing context:

- massage: diluted with a vegetable oil
- inhalation: in a bowl of hot water, as a nebulizer, on a tissue, via a room fragrancer
- in a bath: 3–6 drops, soaking for at least 10 minutes

- as a compress
- in wound care
- mouth-rinses.

Massage

This is a common form of administration since the beneficial effects of touch in combination with appropriate essential oils provide a supportive form of treatment for a variety of problems. Massage can be given to the whole body or to parts, as time permits. Professional training in massage and aromatherapy ensures the correct choice of essential oils and their dilutions in vegetable carrier oils, and appropriate massage techniques. In massage, oils absorbed into the blood-stream via the skin have a systemic effect (Balacs 1992, Jäger et al 1992)

Inhalation

Inhalation of oils affects the body, as the olfactory nerve fibres are directly linked with the limbic system of the brain, the emotional centre (Mosby 1983). Odours affect mood and can prompt memory of past events, happy or sad, so choice of oils is important. Inhalation also takes place when the oils are given via other routes. The essential oils of eucalyptus (*Eucalyptus radiata* ssp. *radiata*) or benzoin (*Styrax benzoe*) have been used by nurses for respiratory inhalations for many years. A drop of true lavender (*Lavandula angustifolia* ssp. *angustifolia*) on a tissue has been reported by nurses to assist sleep in the elderly, confirming some laboratory experiments (Guillemain et al 1989).

Compresses

Compresses with added essential oils can help to relieve pain, such as a warm compress on the abdomen for menstrual pain, or a cold compress on the head may help relieve a bursting headache.

Wound care

Essential oils have a vital role in wound care; for example, the essential oil of tea tree (*Melaleuca alternifolia terpineol-4*), known for its anti-fungal and antiviral effects, has been used in the care of fungating cancer wounds with good effect as well as for more superficial skin lesions such as underneath the breasts of healthy patients (author's personal experience).

Mouth-rinses

For patients receiving chemotherapy, a diluted mouthwash of essential oils including lavender and geranium has been found beneficial for the relief of mouth ulcers in chemotherapy units (author's personal experience).

Therapeutic potential in nursing

Essential oils can be used for a wide range of conditions including:
- stress, anxiety and depression
- insomnia and restlessness
- acute asthma attacks and other respiratory conditions
- common colds and influenza
- digestive disorders, constipation
- muscular and neuralgic pain
- arthritis
- menstrual irregularities, thrush
- headaches and migraine
- burns, eczema, psoriasis and a variety of other skin conditions
- wound and scar healing

Contraindications for use

- If essential oils are administered with massage, then the contraindications for massage apply
- Essential oils must always be diluted before applying to the skin; the dilution will depend on the particular essential oil used and the age, size and condition of the patient
- Sensitive patients or those with allergies should be treated with caution: if in doubt a simple patch test with the proposed blend of oils should be applied, before proceeding with full massage
- Oils for inhalation via fragrancers should be selected for individual patients rather than a whole ward
- Toxicity and contraindications for each oil must be well understood (Tisserand & Balacs 1995)
- Keep essential oils away from eyes and mucous membranes
- In pregnancy, many oils may be contraindicated due to toxic risk to mother and fetus or risk of spontaneous abortion. These include: aniseed, armoise (mugwort), arnica, basil, camomile (avoid in first trimester as it can induce menstruation), camphor, cedar, cinnamon, clary sage, clove, cypress, fennel, hyssop, jasmine, juniper, lavender (*Lavandula stoechas* not at any time; *L. angustifolia* ssp. *angustifolia* not during the first trimester), marjoram, myrrh, niaouli, origanum, pennyroyal, peppermint, sage, savory, rose, rosemary, ravensara, thuja, thyme and wintergreen. Fennel can be used as a tea for morning sickness, but do not use the essential oil (Franchomme & Pénoël 1990, Tisserand & Balacs 1995). New information is now coming to light which may mean that this list may be modified (Guba

Contraindications for use (Cont'd)

1998). Until this is confirmed by other leaders in aromatherapy, it is doubtful that practice will change

- Many of the oils just listed are toxic and not recommended for general use; oils that can be toxic for babies and young children include aniseed, hyssop, some eucalyptus, peppermint, fennel, myrrh, niaouli, camphor, ravensara, sage, thuja
- Do not use oils that elicit a negative psychological response from the patient (ask them)
- Due to the strong association that smell can have with memory, special care should be taken with patients undergoing chemotherapy or those feeling very unwell or sensitive; the smell of the same oil in a subsequent context could induce nausea, vomiting or negative emotions
- Aromatherapy is not for dabblers – undergo professional training before treating patients. There are now several aromatherapy courses available for nurses at university level with additional English National Board accreditation. Find a course appropriate for

Summary

The use of aromatherapy in nursing practice has developed enormously over recent years. The benefits of essential oils have been known for centuries. Good practice requires sound knowledge of the chemical properties of essential oils and their therapeutic indications and contraindications. Safety in the use of essential oils has become the watchword of the 1990s. New evidence is required to disperse some of the fears that have developed in hospitals and other clinical settings. In addition, practical experience is needed to apply aromatherapy appropriately in nursing. Further nursing and chemical research on aromatherapy in the clinical setting will improve understanding of this useful form of complementary therapy. Understanding of essential oils is growing at a rapid rate around the world and it is anticipated that this will continue to develop and change nursing practice in this field.

REFERENCES

Arcier M 1990 Aromatherapy. Hamlyn, London
Balacs T 1992 Dermal crossing. International Journal of Aromatherapy 4: 23–25
Blackwell A L 1991 Tea tree oil and anaerobic (bacterial) vaginosis (Letter). Lancet 337, 300

Buckle J 1993 Does it matter which lavender oil is used? Nursing Times 89: 32–35

Chambers 1988 Chambers English Dictionary. Chambers, Cambridge

Corner J Cawley N Hildebrand S 1995 An evaluation of the use of massage and essential oils on the wellbeing of cancer patients. International Journal of Palliative Nursing 1: 67–73

Dale A Cornwall S 1994 The role of lavender oil in relieving perineal discomfort following childbirth: a blind randomised clinical trial. Journal of Advanced Nursing 19: 89–96

Dunn C 1992 A report on a randomised controlled trial to evaluate the use of massage and aromatherapy in an intensive care unit. Battle Hospital, Reading, unpublished

Evans B 1995 An audit into the effects of aromatherapy massage and the cancer patient in palliative and terminal care. Complementary Therapies in Medicine 3: 239–241

Fowler P Wall M 1997 COSHH and CHIPS: ensuring the safety of aromatherapy. Complementary Therapies in Medicine 5: 112–115

Fowler P Wall M 1998 Aromatherapy: Control of Substances Hazardous to Health. Complementary Therapies in Medicine 6: 85–93

Franchomme P Pénoël D 1990 L'aromathérapie exactement. Roger Jallois, Limoges

Guba R 1998 Toxicity myths: the actual risk of essential oil use (in press)

Guillemain J Rousseau A Delaveau P 1989 Neurodepressive effects of the essential oil of *Lavandula angustifolia* Mill. (French) Annales Pharmaceutiques Françaises 47: 337–343

Hudson R 1996 The value of lavender for rest and activity in the elderly patient. Complementary Therapies in Medicine 4: 52–57

Jäger W Buchbauer G Jirovetz L 1992 Percutaneous absorption of lavender oil from massage oil. Journal of the Society of Cosmetic Chemistry 43: 49–54

Mosby C V 1983 Mosby's medical and nursing dictionary. CV Mosby, St Louis, USA

Stevensen C J 1994 The psychophysiological effects of aromatherapy following cardiac surgery. Complementary Therapies in Medicine 2: 27–35

Tisserand R 1980 The art of aromatherapy. CW Daniels, Saffron Walden, UK

Tisserand R 1998/9 Editorial comment. International Journal of Aromatherapy 9 (2): 49

Tisserand R, Balacs T 1995 Essential oil safety: a guide for health care professionals. Churchill Livingstone, Edinburgh.

Valnet J 1990 The practice of aromatherapy. CW Daniels, Saffron Walden, UK

Wilkinson S 1995 Aromatherapy and massage in palliative care. International Journal of Palliative Nursing 1: 21–30

Williams D 1989 Lecture notes on essential oils. Eve Taylor, London

FURTHER READING – JOURNALS

Avis A 1999 When is an aromatherapist not an aromatherapist? Complementary Therapies in Medicine 7 (2): 116–118

Baker S 1997 Formation and development of the Aromatherapy Organisations Council. Complementary Therapies in Nursing and Midwifery. 3 (3): 78–80

Cannard G 1996 The effect of aromatherapy in promoting relaxation and stress reduction in the general hospital. Complementary Therapies in Nursing and Midwifery 2 (2): 38–40

Cawthorn A 1995 A review of the literature surrounding the research into aromatherapy. Complementary Therapies in Nursing and Midwifery 1 (4): 118–120

Kacperek L 1997 Patients' views on the factors which would influence the use of an aromatherapy massage outpatient service. Complementary Therapies in Nursing and Midwifery 3 (2): 51–57

Stevensen C J 1998 Aromatherapy in dermatology. Clinics in Dermatology 16 (6): 692–694

Styles J 1997 The use of aromatherapy in hospitalised children with HIV disease. Complementary Therapies in Nursing and Midwifery 3(1): 16–20

Tiran D 1996 Aromatherapy and midwifery: Benefits and risks. Complementary Therapies in Nursing and Midwifery 2(4): 88–92

FURTHER READING – BOOKS

Buckle J 1997 Clinical aromatherapy in nursing. Arnold, London

Price S, Price L 1995 Aromatherapy for health professionals. Churchill Livingstone, Edinburgh

Stevensen C J 1996 In: Micozzi M (ed) Fundamentals of complementary and alternative medicine. Churchill Livingstone, New York

Vickers A 1996 Massage and aromatherapy: a guide for health professionals. Chapman and Hall, London

USEFUL ADDRESSES

Aromatherapy Organisations Council (AOC)
3 Laymers Close
Braybrooke,
Market Harborough, Leicester LE16 8LN
Tel/fax: 01858 434242

International Federation of Aromatherapists (IFA)
Department of Continuing Education
Royal Masonic Hospital
Ravenscourt Park
London W6 0TN
Tel: 0181 846 8066

International Society for Professional Aromatherapists (ISPA)
41 Leicester Road
Hinckley
Leicestershire LE10 1LW
Tel: 01455 637 987

Register of Qualified Aromatherapists
54a Gloucester Avenue
London NW1 8JD

17 Autogenic therapy

Dorothy Crowther

Autogenic therapy – a psychophysiological form of psychotherapy, which the patient carries out himself by using passive concentration upon certain combinations of psychophysiologically adapted verbal stimuli Luthe (1963)

Autogenic therapy is not simply another relaxation method. The patient becomes a passive observer in the autogenic state (altered state of consciousness) while the brain's self-regulatory mechanism functions normally, thus allowing homoeostasis (rebalancing) to take place. Over 80 physiological changes have been measured during autogenic practice, demonstrating that a normalizing process takes place (BAFATT 1993).

The technique is easy to learn as it involves simple mental exercises that can be carried out anywhere, in an airport longue, travelling by train, at work, and so on. Unlike many other therapies, autogenic therapy is not reliant upon a therapist; it is a self-empowering tool that once learned can be used whenever required. An adaptable technique, it is ideal for nurses to teach to patients, provided they have the contact time.

HISTORICAL BACKGROUND

Autogenic therapy was developed in Germany in the 1920s by the neuropsychiatrist Dr Johannes Schultz, after observing the work of Professor Oscar Vogt, an eminent researcher on psychophysiological changes of different states of conscious control (known as prophylactic rest periods). Shultz recognized the benefit of prophylactic rest periods to psychiatric patients and this led him to develop the standard exercises that provide the framework of autogenic training.

The original method was extended when Shultz met Dr Wolfgang Luthe in 1940. Research on specific problems in psychiatric patients led Luthe to design techniques complementary to the standard exercises of autogenic therapy (Luthe & Schulz 1969). Dr Luthe left Germany for Canada where he continued work on autogenic therapy. In 1960, he introduced the concept of autogenic neutralization for those who required more than the standard exercises. This involved a consistently longer period in the autogenic state and was, according to Coleman (1988), intended to help psychiatric patients reach a 'curative' state of mental equilibrium. The extent of Luthe's work is seen in six volumes on autogenic therapy and its applications (see Further Reading – Books). Luthe's dedication to autogenic therapy led him to establish research centres in Canada and Japan and there are estimated to be over 3000 scientific papers on autogenic training (Crocker & Grozelle 1991, Kaufman et al 1988).

In 1979, Dr Carruthers and his wife Vera Diamond, a psychotherapist, went to Canada to learn autogenic therapy. They recognized the benefits of this therapy for those at risk from stress-related illness and, in 1980, introduced autogenic training to Britain. In 1984, the British Association of Autogenic Training and Therapy (BAFATT) (now British Autogenic Society 1999) was set up for the regulation of training, maintaining professional standards and promoting research.

TREATMENT

Since autogenic therapy can have a profound effect on an individual, careful assessment and screening must take place. Usually, the patient is interviewed by the trainer to find out why they wished to learn autogenic therapy, since the work requires full cooperation. A full medical history covering physical, psychological, social and spiritual well-being is taken. A letter and a short medical questionnaire are also given to the patient to take to their General Practitioner; this informs the doctor that their patient wishes to undertake autogenic therapy and the returned questionnaire gives the trainer relevant medical information (with the patient's permission).

This method can be taught in small groups of four to six people or individually, depending upon the patient's preference; both methods are effective and streamlined according to individual need. Autogenic therapy requires eight weekly sessions with two follow-up sessions. Each session lasts for 1 hour and, between sessions, patients are expected to practise three times a day and keep a diary of each session. The diary is essential as it provides the trainer with information on the patient's progress, without which therapy cannot continue.

At the start of the therapy the patient is shown how to carry out a body check; this simply means making sure they are comfortable, for example, being aware of any tension and trying to let it go and, if sitting in a chair, ensuring that their feet touch the ground. 'Cancelling out' of the exercise is also taught to ensure that patients can stop whenever they want and are not dependent on the trainer; cancellation is done at the end of each exercise.

The standard exercises are then taught, starting with the heaviness exercise, which is practised by the patient over 7 days, before the other exercise are introduced one at a time over the 8 weeks. During this time the trainer also adds, where appropriate, intentional exercises; these are cathartic and designed to help the patient deal with emotional problems. In addition, a partial exercise is taught for use outside the standard session whenever the need arises; for example, when experiencing a panic attack.

Two follow-up sessions are held at 6 weeks and 3 months after completion of the standard exercises. Patients are advised to contact the trainer during these periods if they have any problems with the method. When first learning the technique a person may experience memories of events long past, such as old injuries. This is normal and occurs only during the exercise; with more experience of the method, it is common to feel heaviness and warmth in the limbs as well as a general feeling of deep relaxation during the exercises.

Stages of technique

The first of the weekly sessions consists of the following stages:

- interview/assessment of client
- introduction to autogenic therapy including body check, cancellation technique and first standard heaviness exercise – dominant arm.

Follow-up weekly sessions are as follows:

- autogenic therapy check
- heaviness of arms and legs
- heaviness of neck and shoulders, partial exercise and peace formulae
- warmth of arms and legs plus introduction to intentional exercises
- heart beat
- breathing
- solar plexus
- forehead
- introduction to space exercise and personal motivation formulae

Therapeutic potential in nursing

Autogenic therapy is a unique relaxation technique that can be used in a variety of health care settings both as a preventive medicine and for improving quality of life for those with illness. Its benefits include:

- deep relaxation
- stress reduction
- pain management

Therapeutic potential in nursing (Cont'd)

- controlling anticipatory nausea/vomiting (in patients undergoing chemotherapy/radiotherapy treatment)
- improving confidence
- controlling/getting rid of panic attacks
- improving sleeping patterns
- integrating awareness of mind and body
- hypertension, etc.

Contraindications for use

Not everyone is suited to autogenic therapy, in particular:

- children under 5 years
- those with no motivation
- people with a personality disorder
- patients with acute psychoses

In some instances, it is important for the patient to be under medical supervision during the training, notably in cases of:

- unstable epilepsy
- insulin-dependent diabetes
- chronic psychoses.

Those who have used unprescribed drugs (e.g. LSD) may also be unsuitable.

Summary

Autogenic therapy has great potential for use by nurses, particularly those working in the primary care sector, i.e. Health Visitors/District Nurses/Practice Nurses and nurses involved in caring for patients with chronic/terminal illness. Training to teach the method takes 2 years and applicants must have undertaken autogenic training themselves and become proficient in self-use for at least 3 months after the course (approximately 9 months in total). All applicants must hold a qualification in one of the health care professions, e.g. medicine, nursing. A list of qualified registered therapists is available from The British Association for Autogenic Training and Therapy (BAFATT) (now British Autogenic Society 1999).

REFERENCES

British Autogenic Society 1999, Autogenic Therapy Brochure. British Autogenic Society, London

BAFATT 1993 Autogenic training information leaflet. BAFATT, London

Coleman J 1988 Luthe's cathartic autogenic training: a therapist's handbook. BAFATT, London

Crocker P R Grozelle C 1991 Journal of Sports Medicine and Physical Fitness 31 (2): 277–282

Freedman R R et al 1991 Psychosomatic medicine. American Psychosomatic Society

Kaufman K L Olson R Tarnowski J K 1989 Self-regulation treatment to reduce the aversiveness of cancer chemotherapy. Journal of Adolescent Health Care (USA) 4: 323–327

Luthe W 1963 Journal of the Hillside Hospital, New York 12 (2): 106–121

Luthe W 1970 Autogenic therapy: research and theory. Grune & Stratton, New York, vol 4

Luthe W Schultz J H 1969 Autogenic therapy. Grune & Stratton, London, vol 1

FURTHER READING – JOURNALS

Crowther D 1991 Complementary therapy in practice. Nursing Standard 5: 25–27

Faulkner A 1990 Autogenics – neighbourhood venture. Nursing Times 86: 50–52

Research in autogenic training is ongoing and has resulted in numerous papers of which abstracts are available in English through the Medline database.

FURTHER READING – BOOKS

Baudouin C 1921 Suggestion and autosuggestion. George Allen & Unwin, London

Kermani K 1990 Autogenic training: the effective holistic way to better health. Souvenir Press, London

Luthe W 1970 Autogenic therapy: dynamics of autogenic neutralisation. Grune & Stratton, New York, vol 5

Luthe W 1973 Autogenic therapy: treatment with autogenic neutralisation. Grune & Stratton, New York, vol 6

Luthe W Schultz J H 1969 Autogenic therapy. Grune & Stratton, New York, vols 1, 2, 3

Pelletier K P 1982 Mind as healer, mind as slayer: a holistic approach to preventing stress disorders. Allen & Unwin, London, p 227–244

USEFUL ADDRESSES

The registered training body is:

The British Autogenic Society
Royal London Homœopathic
Hospital
Great Ormond Street
London WC1N 3HR

Centre for Autogenic Training
Wirral Holistic Care Services
St Catherine's Hospital
Church Road
Birkenhead
Wirral CH42 0LQ

18 Biofeedback

David Bray

Biofeedback – *a method of training which enables a person, mostly with the help of electronic equipment, to learn to control otherwise involuntary bodily functions – 'learning to play the internal organs'*
Lang (1979)

The word biofeedback has been defined as 'information about the state of biological processes, and is used to describe any technique which increases the ability of a person to voluntarily control physiological activities by being provided with information about those activities' (Olton & Noonberg 1980). Biofeedback mostly uses electronic instruments which, when connected to an individual, can measure, amplify and display involuntary physiological processes on a moment to moment basis (Patel 1988). It works on the basic principle that feedback of information, or knowledge of results, is essential for the efficient learning of any skill. The skill in this instance is the control of a given physiological activity, such as heart rate. The information, or knowledge, is the ongoing level of that activity. By monitoring someone's heart rate, for example, and presenting this information to them in a sensible form, such as a digital display, control of the heart rate can be learned (Hume 1976). If such activity is part of a disorder which is not entirely the result of irreversible organic pathology, the trainee can then learn to change the levels of the activity and restore normal function.

The process of biofeedback can be seen as a feedback loop, as shown in Figure 18.1. The level of activity of a 'target organ' is picked up by an instrument, which produces signals presented to the trainee through the senses (sight, sound or other). These are then interpreted by the trainee at the conscious level (brain). The appropriate state of mind or bodily sensations which either increase or decrease activity levels are then identified and enhanced by the trainee to modify the activity of the target organ. A target organ can be any body part from which changing levels of activity can be demonstrated, directly or indirectly, for example skin, muscle, brain, heart, blood vessels, respiratory system. Feedback from a particular target organ is often

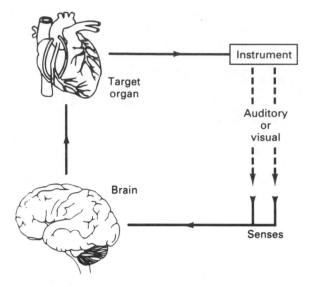

Figure 18.1 *The biofeedback loop.*

used to affect other functions; for example in influencing essential hypertension by modifying skin resistance.

HISTORICAL BACKGROUND

For several hundred years, there have been reports from India of yogis who could slow their heart beat, increase their body temperature, survive with little oxygen (reduce their metabolic rate) and influence other bodily functions not normally under voluntary control. However, those capable of this control underwent rigorous and lengthy training, usually in a religious context, and the reports failed to suggest techniques that could be effectively taught to a large percentage of unselected individuals (Barber 1970). More recently, control of involuntary functions has been achieved using hypnosis, autogenic training, and spontaneously in a few rare individuals (Green et al 1970). Using electronic instruments to provide direct readings of levels of involuntary activities has led to a range of effective techniques, representing a synthesis of ancient skills and modern technology.

One of the first recorded successful uses of biofeedback instrumentation was by the Russian psychologist Lisina in 1958, involving taught control of vascular constriction and dilatation (Gatchel & Price 1979). There has been an explosion of research into biofeedback since then, and it is estimated that over 3000 journal articles and 100 books have been published. Many early research findings were disputed due to faulty methodology, but biofeedback is increasingly accepted and Schwartz (1987) suggests it has come of age.

TREATMENT

Biofeedback instruments

These are often called machines but this is not strictly correct, as a machine is something that performs work. However, the instruments used in biofeedback do not *do anything to* people. They are measuring devices, and only provide information about fluctuating activity levels of target organs. In this respect, biofeedback instruments should be seen as teaching aids only, and are no longer needed once the trainee has learned the skill. Instruments are designed according to the target organ activity to be monitored. Any electrical current applied to the skin is not felt by the trainee, and mains-powered equipment has built-in safety features to avoid potentially dangerous direct contact with mains electricity:

- Skin resistance/conductivity monitors (galvanic skin response – GSR; electrodermal response – EDR): register general levels of autonomic arousal; activity increases during 'tension' and reduces during relaxation.
- Skin temperature monitors: register skin temperature changes related to vasodilation/vasoconstriction, which is an indication of the stress response in some people, and is also important in some peripheral vascular disorders. A simplified version is the use of strips or 'dots' of thermoreactive material which adhere to the skin, changing colour with skin temperature changes, e.g. black when tense, blue when relaxed ('Biodots' – see Useful Addresses). Unless the user is properly informed, this material could be very misleading, since some people do not exhibit skin temperature changes when tense, and the environmental temperature must be within a certain constant range when the material is used. Within these limitations, they are useful aids for relaxation training, some peripheral vascular disorders and migraine headaches.
- Myographic (EMG) monitors: provide a direct indication of activity in accessible muscles, and can be used to enhance muscle activity, as in recovery after cerebrovascular accident (CVA) or to reduce electrical activity in muscles when there is too much activity (muscular tension) in the resting state, and bring about effective muscular relaxation
- Electroencephalographic (EEG) monitors: register brain wave activity, enabling trainees to generate wave forms such as alpha

waves, associated with a relaxed state. Systems have been designed whereby the desired wave forms enable a model electric train to move round a track.

- Heart/pulse rate or rhythm monitors.

Computer-enhanced biofeedback

Computerized systems are available which enable records to be kept at any stage of the training process, in the form of graphs. These records can be printed out. The computerized system can also make learning more fun. The signal of activity levels is used as a control for computer games. For example, tensing and releasing the frontalis muscle to guide a ship through a channel on the computer screen can help tension headache (Myolink system and Myostart programme, Aleph One Ltd – see Useful Addresses).

The training method

During a biofeedback session, the trainee sits or lies comfortably in relatively quiet surroundings (earphones can be used for auditory feedback, or to reduce distracting background noise). Comfortable electrodes are attached to clean skin. The anatomical location of the electrodes depends on which target organ or type of instrument is used: for general electrodermal response, usually around two fingers; for muscle activity, to the skin near the muscle origin and insertion; for temperature regulation, to the skin of hands or feet; and for EEG activity, to the cranial area. The trainee spends sessions of 15–40 minutes practising with the instrument. The total number of sessions needed will vary from person to person, depending upon the nature of the problem, and the degree of compliance (from 4 to 20 sessions). As with training in any kind of skill, there will be individual differences in initial capacities for learning and learning rates. Sessions may take place several times per week and continue from a few weeks to a few months. Once the trainee has been shown what to do, the continued presence of the trainer is not needed, as the trainee continues to learn on their own with the aid of the instrument.

Stages of technique

First contact – explanation. The most important aspect of biofeedback is *learning* on the part of the trainee, who should be well-informed about the concepts, aims and process of training. General considerations are that biofeedback involves the learning of a skill, is not an instant answer, will take time and practice, and that any problems that arise should be recognized and discussed with the

Stages of technique (Cont'd)

trainer. The key factors for success are high motivation and compliance on the part of the trainee.

Initial session/s with the instrument – familiarization. The main aim of the first session is for the trainee to become familiar with the equipment. To most people, biofeedback is a strange and unusual experience and a gradual introduction to the process is sometimes necessary. The trainee finds out how the target organ levels change with alterations in movement, breathing and mental activity. By mutual agreement with the trainer, the trainee is then shown (if necessary) which accessory relaxation techniques, or other methods, to use to enhance the biofeedback process.

Follow-up sessions – practice. Trainees continue to practise on their own. Some briefing or debriefing with the trainer may be needed occasionally.

Completion of training. Training is complete when the trainee is able to self-regulate without the instrumentation.

Therapeutic potential in nursing

Therapeutic benefit depends upon the instruments (and time) available to the nurse, the level of expertise and the environment. The needs of patients in a community clinic differ from those of hospital inpatients. The type of department in a hospital determines which kind of biofeedback is appropriate. For the beginner, a GSR/EDR monitor is perhaps the first step, since it is less expensive, portable, versatile and easily applied. Conscientious reading and study are essential for basic knowledge and further progress. General applications include:

- Demonstrating to patients that tension is related to mental activity, and that they are capable of developing some control of tension levels
- Rapidly and effectively teaching patients to relax/release tension, including enhancing and accelerating the effects of autogenic therapy, hypnosis, meditation-based relaxation and progressive muscular relaxation (biofeedback instruments let trainees know clearly and quickly when they are doing the right thing)
- Pain control
- Observing whether or not an anxious patient (injured, preoperative, prepartum, etc.) is 'calming down'.

Biofeedback can also be used to influence behaviour (see contraindications):

- by reducing anxiety levels in phobic patients
- by assisting in reducing tension as part of weight control and in substance dependency.

It can contribute to the management of specific conditions (but see contraindications) such as:

Therapeutic potential in nursing (Cont'd)

- asthma
- cardiovascular disorders (arrhythmias, hypertension, recovery from coronary episode)
- headache (migraine and tension)
- insomnia
- neuromuscular problems (rehabilitation, spasticity, paralysis (especially after CVA), muscular tension)
- peripheral vascular disorders.

A prospective biofeedback trainer should (ideally) have the following:

- Some technical ability in order to apply and maintain the instruments
- Good communication, counselling and teaching skills
- Knowledge of a variety of relaxation/stress management techniques which can be used to supplement biofeedback training
- Some ability to understand and control their own stress responses.

Contraindications for use

People who are repelled by instruments/computers (this is also a contraindication for would-be trainers), who see no possibility of having any control over what happens to them, or who have very low self-esteem, are not suitable candidates. The Biofeedback Standards Association's 'Applications, standards and guidelines' (Schwartz & Fehmi 1982) is suggested as essential reading for any prospective trainer and includes the following 'cautions and contraindications':

- A variety of psychiatric disorders, including severe depression
- Impairment of attention/memory, as in dementia or mental handicap
- Anyone experiencing a severe health or emotional crisis
- Low blood pressure
- Seizure disorders
- Extreme scepticism.

Relative contraindications apply when patients are receiving medication for certain conditions such as asthma, glaucoma and diabetes mellitus (Schwartz 1987). The patient's physician should be consulted, and medication doses monitored if biofeedback training is used. Where possible, training should be part of multidisciplinary health care.

Biofeedback training using instrumentation is ideally suited to the busy nurse who may have a reasonable amount of time available to teach self-help techniques to patients. The method enables people to take an active part in their own recovery. It is non-invasive and fosters self-reliance, independence and responsibility for improvement in health.

In the late 1990s, much work has been done to confirm effectiveness, and expand applications of biofeedback (Journal of Applied Psychophysiology and Biofeedback). In addition to the conditions listed above, thermal Biofeedback has been used in the treatment of irritable bowel syndrome, neurocardiogenic syncope, and migraine ('Warm hands mean a cool, quiet head'). EMG biofeedback has been utilized in incontinence (strengthening the muscles of the pelvic floor), and carpal tunnel syndrome. One case study describes improvement of 'Split stretch' in a healthy gymnast!

The medium which has been given most attention is EEG (Evans & Abarbanel, 1999). Benefits have been reported in learning difficulties, addiction, attention deficit, brain injury, hyperactivity, and identity disorder. Of particular interest is the use of EEG in 'locked in' syndrome, where a person suffering from motor neurone disease or brain stem stroke is totally paralysed while sight and hearing remain intact. Individuals have been taught to control brain wave patterns to activate an alphabet board, so enabling them to communicate (Birbaumer & Ghanayim 1999). The use of EEG biofeedback, not only for self-regulation, but in its potential for control of machines and vehicles, promises very exciting developments for the future.

REFERENCES

Barber T X 1970 In: Stoyva J et al (eds) Biofeedback and self-control. Aldine Atherton, Chicago

Birnbaumer N Ghanayim N et al 1999 Spelling device for the paralysed. Nature 398: 297–298

Gatchel R J Price K P (eds) 1979 Clinical applications of biofeedback: appraisal and status. Pergamon, New York

Green E Green A Walters M 1970 Voluntary control of internal states: physiological and psychological. In: Stoyva J et al (eds) Biofeedback and self-control. Aldine Atherton, Chicago

Hume W I 1976 Biofeedback. Annual Research Review. Eden Press, Lancaster, vol 2

Journal of Applied Psychophysiology and Biofeedback 1997–1999, vols 22–24, Plenum Press, New York

Lang P J 1979 In: Gatchel R J Price K P (eds) Clinical applications of biofeedback: appraisal and status. Pergamon, New York

Olton D S Noonberg A R 1980 Biofeedback – clinical applications in behavioural medicine. Prentice Hall, Englewood Cliffs, New Jersey

Patel C 1988 Biofeedback and self-regulation. In: Rankin-Box D F (ed) Complementary health therapies: a guide for nurses and the caring professions. Croom Helm, Beckenham, Kent

Schwartz M S 1987 Biofeedback – a practitioner's guide. Guilford Press, New York

Schwartz M S Fehmi L 1982 Applications, standards and guidelines for providers of biofeedback services. Biofeedback Society of America (see AAPB below)

FURTHER READING – JOURNALS

Biofeedback and Self-Regulation – published quarterly by Plenum, New York
Patel C Marmot M M Terry D J 1981 Controlled trial of biofeedback-aided
behavioural methods in reducing mild hypertension. British Medical
Journal 282: 2005–2008
Biofeedback research is published in a wide variety of contexts and lack of
space prohibits a detailed list – other journal references can be found in the
above references.

FURTHER READING – BOOKS

Basmajian J V 1983 Biofeedback: principles and practice for clinicians.
Williams & Wilkins, Baltimore
Brown B 1977 Stress and the art of biofeedback. Harper & Row, New York
Evans J R Abarbanel 1999 Introduction to quantitative EEG and
neurofeedback, Academic Press, San Diego
Hume W I 1977 Biofeedback. Annual Research Review. Eden Press, Lancaster,
vol 2
Stoyva J et al (eds) 1972 on (annuals) Biofeedback and self-control. Aldine
Atherton, Chicago

USEFUL ADDRESSES

Because biofeedback instruments do not change patients, but only supply
information to encourage people to be self-caring, they are safe and unlikely
to cause harm. Currently there is no standardized training in Britain, and no
central register. However, the addresses cited here are sources of national
information.

Association of Applied
Psychophysiology and Biofeedback
10200 West 44th Ave #304
Wheat Ridge
CO 80033, USA

International Stress Management
Association (UK Branch)
South Bank University LPSS
103 Borough Rd
London SE1 0AA

British Holistic Medical Association
179 Gloucester Place
London NW1 6DX

Biofeedback instrument suppliers:

Aleph One Ltd
The Old Court House
High Street

Bottisham
Cambridge CB5 9BB
Tel: 01223 811679

(also an excellent source of
publications on research and
practical applications)

Biodata Ltd 10 Stocks Street
Manchester M8 8QG
Tel: 0161 834 6688

Biodots
Stresswise
Department of Biological Science
Manchester Metropolitan
University
John Dalton Building
Chester Street
Manchester M1 5GD

19 Bach Flower Remedies

Ruth Benor

Bach Flower Remedies – *The use of flower essences to promote emotional equilibrium.*
'True healing involves treating the very base of the cause of the suffering. Therefore no effort directed to the body alone can do more than superficially repair the damage. Treat people for their emotional unhappiness, allow them to be happy, and they will become well' Dr Edward Bach

Flower remedies or essences are rapidly increasing in popularity, along with other natural remedies from the plant kingdom. Flower essences are amongst the most accessible therapies, are relatively inexpensive, immediately available, easy to use and rarely produce unpleasant side-effects.

The use of flower therapies in health care is driven by the patient population, with increasing interest from health care practitioners rapidly following. For some they are a natural 'drug delivery system' (Hoffman 1996). For others they offer a complementary approach/support for existing orthodox treatments. An esoteric point of view suggests flower essences can be an important aspect of a total healing journey (Hoffman 1996).

Flower remedies are not pharmaceutically processed and do not contain active chemicals. They are not habit-forming, are a non-prescription item and can be bought in health food shops and high street pharmacies. The remedies are thought to work as energy patterning in the water that is used as the delivery medium. Flower blossoms and twigs placed in water leave a vital force pattern that mirrors positive emotions experienced by humans and animals. After the energetic pattern has infused the water with its essence, the blossom is removed from the water and no organic part of the plant remains in the solution. Flower remedies are therefore grouped with other energetic patterning medicines – e.g. homeopathy – as subtle energy, or vibrational medicine.

Resonations between the energetic patterns of the remedies and the emotional patterns of the individual appear to bring about benefits by influencing each person's own life-force (Harvey et al 1995). They provide a natural, self-help therapy designed to aid the person in regaining emotional equilibrium during periods of stress, conflict, or dis-ease or illnesses (Howard 1993).

The Bach Flower Remedies are the best known of the remedies, forerunners to a growing number of flower essence ranges available internationally. Many countries now have their own ranges of remedies.

HISTORICAL BACKGROUND

The Bach Flower Remedies were developed more than 60 years ago by a British physician and homeopath, Edward Bach (pronounced Batch). Bach (1886–1936) was an intuitive, sensitive physician. He became increasingly dissatisfied with the limited focus of orthodox medicine of his time. He saw medical practices reducing the person of the patient to only the component physical parts, with treatment focused mostly on symptoms. Little attention was given to exploring the causes and effects of an illness, or the meaning the illness held for the person as a whole. Bach recognized the importance and influence of the personality characteristics and the influence of attitudes and emotions on any given situation presenting in a physical or emotional challenge. He achieved this insight not only from the vantage of a physician but also as a direct result of his own physical frailties and illnesses.

Bach recognized the importance of the mind, body and spirit in preventing and overcoming illnesses. He considered that dis-ease and illness were the result of inner conflict, manifested in negative states of feeling and thinking. The flower remedies, which carry a positive emotional response, can enable the individual to be freed from their negative emotional states by restoring them to the best qualities of their innate characteristics, and by reconnecting them to their innate healing potential and wholeness.

In the late twentieth century, this awareness has been well developed in the holistic movement, which emphasizes the discernible interconnectedness of mind, emotions, body and spirit. When a person is compromised, by illness or dis-ease, the dysfunctions are not limited to the symptomatic system or part, but affect people at all levels of their being.

The flower remedies take effect by treating the individual and are not intended to directly treat physical illness. The selection of a remedy is always based on an assessment of the individual's personality. The assessment then moves on to identify the issues and their emotional response to the presenting problem. Even in the presence of the same diagnostic condition (such as arthritis, anxiety, or depression), various individuals will react differently, their responses shaped by the way they feel about themselves, their personal, social and environmental history, their coping styles and their attitude towards health and illness.

The remedies are selected to help during times of immediate crisis or illness and during those times when the individual is called upon to deal with more chronic suffering. They can also be used to enhance the states of individuals who consider themselves well but who would like to improve upon what they are already doing to reach optimum health and well-being.

Dr Bach identified 38 emotional states, each of which was then aligned to a single remedy. The remedy states cluster within seven groups, each associated with a fundamental reaction to conflict:

- fear
- uncertainty
- insufficient interest in present circumstances
- loneliness
- over-sensitivity to influences and ideas
- despondency and despair
- over-care for the welfare of others.

Thirty-seven of the remedies are made from infusion of wild flowers, tree blossoms, or twigs and one remedy is taken from a natural spring attributed with healing qualities.

The remedies are in liquid form, taken by mouth. They may be diluted in a drink or dropped straight onto the tongue. The remedies can be taken singly, but often more than one remedy is recommended. As many as six individual remedies can be combined in a treatment bottle. A remedy is taken as four drops from the treatment bottle four times daily, for approximately 3 weeks. The remedies usually do not have the immediate effects we have come to expect from experience with allopathic medicines, and generally work on a cumulative basis over a period of days to months, though some people may have a more rapid response. A single combined remedy may be sufficient but in some instances a series of treatments unfolds over a period of several months, punctuated by periodic consultation with the practitioner.

Rescue Remedy is the best known combination of five single remedies, used to treat states of distress, or emergencies:

■ Star of Bethlehem	*for after effects of shock*
■ Rock Rose	*Terror and panic*
■ Clematis	*Faintness-feeling out of body with the shock,*
■ Cherry Plum	*for fear of the mind giving way, desperation*
■ Impatiens	*irritability, stress and tension*

Rescue Remedy is available in the usual liquid form and is the only composite remedy also available in cream to be used on the skin. In the topical form it includes a sixth remedy, Crab Apple, for cleansing and smoothing.

TREATMENT

Dr Bach intended the remedies to be used by the individual without having to rely upon a practitioner. By identifying how they are feeling and by referring to the plethora of books on the remedies, one can self-treat. However, to be truly objective about one's own condition, and to distinguish the precise nature of a condition, is difficult. For these reasons it is often more helpful to seek the consultation of a trained Bach Flower practitioner.

After a detailed assessment the practitioner will have a two-fold focus in selecting the remedies. The first is to establish the basic and fundamental nature of the person, in order to find their *remedy type*. This must be incorporated in the treatment remedy. The second is to identify the negative mood or emotional states that are presenting, either as part of the basic personality characteristics, or those that have arisen out of character and are in response to stressful issues or problems.

Remedies may have a spectrum of functions. For instance, Scleranthus is given to people who have difficulty in making up their minds, but it is also a useful remedy for those who have irregular or fluctuating moods or lack consistency in their confidence to make a final decision.

Chestnut Bud is given to those who have difficulty in learning from previous mistakes, or where there is a problem in staying aware of self-perpetuating issues. An example might be the habitual dieter who alternates between eating and not eating. This remedy can help to learn the importance of eating for health rather than repeatedly excluding food only to resort to overeating when feeling stressed by excluding food.

During times of illness or loss, the combination of Star of Bethlehem and Sweet Chestnut remedies can make a significant contribution to help the individual to cope with the exhausting demands that acute and chronic or life-threatening illness can bring.

Contraindications for use

People taking Antabuse or any other medicine designed to stop recovering alcoholics drinking should take medical advice before using Bach Flower Remedies; this is because of the alcohol in the stock bottle. Otherwise the amount of alcohol taken is so small that it can be

Contraindications for use (Cont'd)

disregarded. However, some recovering alcoholics, not on Antabuse, prefer external use to avoid the psychological effects of breaking a commitment not to drink. The remedies can also be made using cider vinegar if necessary.

Therapeutic potential in nursing

- The effects of the remedies do not rely on the individual's belief in them to be effective (Ramsell 1991)
- Remedies are safe for babies and young children (Howard 1994)
- Remedies are used to treat animals and plants (Ball 1999a.).

Stages of technique

Sun infusion preparation method
- Fresh healthy flowers are picked soon after they come into bloom
- Blossom is floated in spring water, left out in the sunshine for 3–4 hours
- The flowers are removed
- The energized essence is mixed with equal volume of brandy to form the mother tincture or flower stock. The brandy acts as a preservative
- Remedies are distributed in 10-ml brown glass dropper bottles
- Shelf-life is 5 years.

Directions on how to make up a remedy

Put two drops from each single remedy in bottle

The bottle should have a 30 ml capacity

Fill up with spring water

Take 4 drops at least 4 times a day.

Summary

Research into the remedies is limited; there are, however, future plans for controlled clinical trails. Bach Flower Remedies are helpful aids to self-care. They offer treatments for many problems. While they are not a panacea for everything in our lives, their contribution is enormous to support and promote health and wholeness.

REFERENCES

Ball S 1999 Bach Flower Remedies for animals. CW Daniel, London
Harvey C Cochrane A 1995 The encyclopaedia of flower remedies. Thorsons, London
Hoffman D 1996 Foreword. In: McIntyre A (ed) The complete floral healer. Gaia Books, London
Howard J 1994 Growing up with Bach Flower Remedies. CW Daniel, London
Ramsell J 1991 Questions and Answers: The Bach Flower Remedies. CW Daniel, London

FURTHER READING – JOURNALS

Bach Flower Remedies

Bach E (reprinted 1993) Heal thysel. CW Daniel, London
Ball S 1999 Principles of Bach Flower Remedies. Thorsons, London
Ball S 1998 The Bach Remedies workbook. CW Daniel, London
Ball S 1996 Bach Flower Remedies for men. CW Daniel, London
Blome G 1999 Advanced Bach flower therapy. Healing Arts Press, Rochester, VT
Chancellor P M 1993 Illustrated handbook of the Bach Flower Remedies. CW Daniel, London
Howard J 1992 Bach Flower Remedies for women. CW Daniels, London
Kramer D Wild H 1996 New Bach Flower body maps. Healing Arts Press, Rochester, VT
Ramsell J 1991 Questions and answers: explaining the basic principles and standards of The Bach Flower Remedies. CW Daniels, London
Scheffer M 1986 Bach Flower therapy: theory and practice. Thorsons, London
Scheffer M 1996 Mastering Bach: a guide to flower diagnosis and treatment therapies. Healing Arts Press, Rochester, VT
Week N 1973 The medical discoveries of Edward Bach. Keats, Connecticut
Weeks N Bullen V 1964 The Bach Flower Remedies: illustrations and preparations. CW Daniel, London

Flower essence therapies

Harvey C Cochrane A 1995 The encyclopaedia of flower remedies: the healing power of flowers from around the world. Thorsons, London
Johnson S 1996 The essence of healing: a guide to the Alaskan flower, gem, and environmental essences. Alaskan Flower Essence Project, Alaska
Kaminski P Katz R 1994 Flower essence repertory: a comprehensive guide to North American and English flower essences for emotional and spiritual well-being. Flower Essence Repertory, Nevada City, CA
Wright-Small M 1988 Flower essences: rendering our understanding and approach to illness and health. Perelandra

USEFUL ADDRESSES

For training seminars, practitioner training, books and remedies, other resources:

The Edward Bach Foundation
Mount Vernon
Sotwell
Oxon OX10 0PZ UK
Tel: 01491 834678

website: www. bachcentre.com
and/or foundation@bachcentre.com

20 Communication skills and counselling

Anne Cawthorn

Counselling skills *– a repertoire of learnt behaviours, both verbal and non-verbal, which enable a rapport to be established between nurse and client and facilitate communication* Evans (1995).

Communication is an essential component of health care. Nurses communicate with clients, relatives and other health professionals, in a range of settings. Verbal and non-verbal communication is the means to understanding and assessing clients. This is, perhaps, of particular importance in complementary medicine, where effective client communication is one way to develop the therapeutic relationship. This is an essential component of a therapy and Mitchell & Cormack (1998) refer to the research on counselling and psychotherapy, which identifies that it may be the experience of the therapeutic relationship in itself that facilitates change in the client. Cawthorn & Billington (1998) refer to the therapeutic relationship as having three components: intimacy, partnership and reciprocity, and through the use of complementary therapies the nurse is communicating acceptance of the patient.

Whilst recognizing the need for good communication, the reality is that it is an area still requiring improvement. Research has demonstrated that patients feel dissatisfied with both the quality of communication and the quantity of information received (Ley 1988). What is said to clients is not understood and frequently forgotten (Reading 1981, Taub & Baker 1983).

Studies by Wilkinson (1991) and Heaven & Maguire (1996) found that nurses use blocking behaviours such as changing the subject, giving premature advice and reassurance. Booth et al (1996) identified that nurses blocked patients' attempts to disclose concerns or express emotions when they were feeling unsupported themselves.

In an attempt to close this communication gap, skills derived from counselling are increasingly being used in nursing. Counselling skills are included in Project 2000 and Bachelor of Nursing programmes and are a component of many post-registration courses. They are also part of many complementary therapy courses and are a pre-requisite to the ENB A49 complementary therapy courses at Manchester Victoria University.

HISTORICAL BACKGROUND

The BAC defines counselling as: 'An interaction in which one person offers another person time, attention, and respect, with the intention of helping that person explore, discover and clarify ways of living more successfully and towards greater well being' (Palmer et al 1996). Stewart (1992) suggests that 'counselling helps clients make some sense out of confusion; choice from conflict and sense out of nonsense'

Historically, counselling draws from a range of theories. These may be broadly divided into:

- Humanistic – Carl Rogers
- Psychoanalytic – Sigmund Freud
- Behavioural – B F Skinner.

Although both psychoanalytic and behavioural theories are used in health care, humanistic theory is most appropriate for nursing interventions. Best known of the humanists are Carl Rogers, the founder of client-centred therapy (Rogers 1961), and Eric Berne who developed Transactional Analysis (popularized through books such as *Games People Play* (Berne 1964) and more recent texts by Ian Stewart (1989, 1996)).

Today many theorists take an integrative approach, drawing from the various skills to formulate a model or framework for practice. Such an approach, frequently encountered in health care, is the helping model of Egan (1995). Egan describes the age-old belief that some people are capable of enabling others to cope with the problems of life. Today, this role falls to counsellors, the clergy, psychiatrists and social workers. In addition to these front-line workers, other professionals who come into contact with, and who are often expected to help with individuals during times of crisis or transition, include health care professionals, nurses and those providing complementary therapies.

As nurses have been increasingly expected to use aspects of counselling in daily practice, it has become important to describe what this entails. There is a difference between professional counselling and the use of the general principles of counselling; much of the nurse–patient relationship falls into the latter category, commonly referred to as 'counselling skills' (Bond 1993). This has been recognized by the British Association of Counselling (BAC 1992) in their code of ethics and practice for counselling skills.

Some nurses and complementary therapists have a recognized counselling qualification and it is acknowledged that on occasions they move temporarily into the role of counsellor. However, Stewart (1992) reminds us that if the need for counselling is perceived it should not be entered into without agreement from both parties. The relationship should be agreed and the roles clearly defined.

If the therapist feels that they are competent to carry out counselling they will need to make this explicit, set a contract and set boundaries. In addition, how this fits in with the complementary therapy will need to be clarified rather than tagging it on to the end of a therapeutic intervention. Mackareth (1999) reminds us that if we find ourselves in this situation we should consider Crossman's 3 Ps:

- protection
- permission
- potency (Crossman 1966).

Protection

- This extends to the therapeutic relationship as well as the practitioner and client. For example, difficulties arising from their work can be taken by counsellors to their regular clinical supervision (CS) meetings. This arrangement is a requirement of their training and ongoing practice. Nurses using complementary therapies may wish to consider engaging in CS to provide protection and support (see chapter 5, clinical supervision).

- The boundaries of confidentiality are also something which need considering in relation to protection. This should ensure protection for both the practitioner and the client. For example whilst it is important to respect a client's confidentiality, there are certain circumstances when information will need to be passed on. Bond (1993) refers to the BAC Code of Ethics (1992) which states that 'counsellors should take all reasonable steps to communicate clearly the extent of confidentiality they are offering to clients'. It goes on to state that if confidentiality needs reviewing this should be done by negotiation between the client and therapist.

Both parties should be aware through establishing the therapeutic boundaries that the contract may need to be renegotiated if the client discloses:

- They are contemplating self-harm, e.g. suicide
- They are contemplating harming others, e.g. murder, child abuse
- They have impaired cognitive ability, e.g. mental illness such as psychosis or are moderately/severely depressed.

If any of the above situations arise, permission may need to be sought from the client so that an appropriate person can be informed. This is usually the client's general practitioner or consultant, although who to contact can be agreed when establishing the contract.

Permission

- Permission needs to be sought if emotional issues are to be explored; this also applies to intimate issues such as relationship and sexual problems. A simple question such as, 'Is it alright to talk about this?' should allow the client to stop if they do not want to pursue a certain issue.

Even when the practitioner has not set out to explore emotional issues, they are occasionally put in a position where they need to handle a cathartic release from the client. Occasionally clients release previously repressed emotions when receiving nurturing touch and support in a safe and therapeutic space. This is more likely to occur when clients are faced with illness and disability, especially when their illness is of a life-threatening nature. Mackereth (1999) recommends that when faced with this situation, one should remain calm and support the client whilst they experience the emotions. If they want to talk about what happened, then empathic listening can be used to facilitate this. Remember that permission should be sought from the client first.

Potency

- All three Ps work together to enable both the practitioner and the client to maximize the healing and helping potential of the therapeutic work. For the practitioner being potent can be developed and supported through effective training and ongoing supervision. Learning is never complete – this acknowledgement can help us as practitioners to continue to explore our skills, pursue professional development and refer on when our boundaries of practice are clear. Receiving feedback from clients, colleagues, teachers and supervisors can also help to assess, develop and appreciate our skills and potency as a practitioner (see chapter 5, Clinical Supervision).

- Potency for the client could be maximized by knowing that their practitioner has had appropriate training and receives ongoing supervision. Having clear boundaries sustained by a contract for the work may provide a space for the client to really be heard and understood. For example, referring on rather than attempting to dabble in dietary advice or psychotherapy.

Buckman (1998) recommends that it is useful to acknowledge emotions using this three-step approach:

1. Identify the emotion
2. Identify the root cause of the emotion
3. Respond in a way that tells you have made the connection between 1 & 2.

An example of this from the author's experience was when a client sobbed every time he received a massage; the touch reminded of him of his mother's, for whom he had not fully grieved. An empathic response that encapsulated this for him was 'you are sad (emotion) because my touch reminds you of your mother who died a long time ago and you still miss her' (root cause). Part of this client's recovery entailed referral to CRUSE for bereavement counselling, as the emotions were those associated with the early stages of grieving which he had not allowed himself to work through.

Effective 'counselling or helping skills'

Most clients do not want formal counselling but benefit from the use of counselling or helping skills. Nelson-Jones (1996) describes a range of helping skills which nurses or complementary therapists use:

- It is a relationship
- It involves a repertoire of skills
- It emphasizes self-help
- It emphasizes choice
- It focuses on problems of living
- It is a process.

When using helping skills the client-centred framework described by Rogers (1980) makes an ideal basis to develop the therapeutic relationship. Roger's four core conditions needed to establish a counselling relationship are:

- empathy
- genuineness
- respect
- Unconditional positive regard.

When these core conditions are present the fundamental counselling relationship exists in which the client may move towards the resolution of problems. In a pure Rogerian framework, the counsellor adopts a non-directive client-centred role. The theory is that, within the therapeutic relationship, clients will be enabled to self-actualize and develop the abilities, latent within themselves, to resolve or accept their situation.

TREATMENT

An awareness of the impact of non-verbal cues is essential in counselling. Non-verbal communication includes:

- clothing and appearance
- use of paralanguage (meaning conveyed by tone and pitch of voice, such as 'uhhu' or hmmm')
- bodily contact and proximity
- respect of personal space
- eye contact
- facial expression.

Generally, counselling skills involve the following:

- accurate listening
- attending
- the use of silence
- appropriate body language
- reflecting, i.e. repeating the client's words to demonstrate listening
- summarizing, i.e. accurately paraphrasing what the client has said
- self-awareness
- use of 'minimal encouragers' or paralanguage.

Listening

This is perhaps the most important skill. Listening can be very therapeutic. For many clients a therapy session is an opportunity to tell their story and be heard. Through active listening the practitioner is being invited to witness their narrative and journey with them as it is unravelled. Tschudin (1995) reminds us that if you know how to listen and what to listen for, you will listen better. She adds, 'listening is active. It is a process, a journey'.

Therapeutic listening has three phases:

- Receiving and understanding
- Communication of your understanding
- An awareness in the other person that you have listened and understood (Van Ooijen & Charnock 1994).

To achieve therapeutic listening the nurse or therapist needs to try and see things from the patient's frame of reference and listen to not only what they are saying but how they are saying it. This requires attention to verbal and non-verbal cues. Both nurses and therapists are in a privileged position where they share an intimate relationship with clients. Below are some ways that counselling skills can be misused.

Contraindications for use

Counselling skills should not be used to:

- Relate one's own similar experience
- Moralize
- Psychoanalyse
- Fantasize about what may be the problem
- Persuade or bully
- Satisfy the nurse's curiosity or needs.

Counselling is not an innate skill but requires careful training and the ability to recognize one's own limitations.

The practitioner should also be aware of the necessity of referring on clients who require specialist help.

Carl Rogers (1980) quotes Lao-tzu:

'If I keep from meddling with people, they take care of themselves,

If I keep from commanding people, they behave themselves,

If I keep from preaching at people, they improve themselves,

If I keep from imposing on people, they become themselves.'

Summary

Whilst not all nurses and complementary therapists may see themselves as effective counsellors, effective communication skills are essential in daily nursing practice. The acquisition of skills drawn from counselling broadens the individual nurse's repertoire of skills leading towards improved client care. The therapeutic value of counselling skills is such that they should form an essential part of training of both the nurse and complementary therapist. The inclusion of clinical supervision should be available to ensure safe and effective practice.

REFERENCES

Berne E 1964 Games people play. Grove Press, New York
Bond T 1993 Counselling, counselling skills and professional roles. In: Bayne R Nicolson P (eds) Counselling and psychotherapy for health professionals. Chapman & Hall, London
Bond T 1993 Standards and ethics for counselling in action. Sage, London
BAC 1992 Code of ethics and practice for counselling skills. British Association for Counselling (BAC), Rugby

Booth K Maguire P Butterworth T Hillier V 1996 Perceived professional support and the use of blocking behaviours by hospice nurses. Journal of Advanced Nursing 24: 522–527

Buckman R 1998 Communication in palliative care: a practical guide. In: Doyle D Hanks G W C MacDonald (eds) Oxford textbook of palliative medicine, 2nd edn. Oxford Medical Publications, Oxford

Bumard P 1992 Effective communication skills for health professionals. Chapman & Hall, London

Cawthorn A Billington 1998 Complementary therapeutic interventions. In: Hill J (ed) Rheumatology nursing: a creative approach. Churchill Livingstone, Edinburgh

Crossman P 1966 Permission and protection. Transactional Analysis Bulletin 5 (19): 152–154

Egan G 1995 The skilled helper: a systematic approach to effective helping, 5th edn. Brooks Cole, CA

Evans E 1995 Communication skills and counselling. In: Rankin-Box D (ed) The Nurses' Handbook of Complementary Therapies, 1st edn. Churchill Livingstone, Edinburgh

Heaven C M Maguire P 1996 Training hospice nurses to elicit patient concerns. Journal of Advanced Nursing 23: 280–286

Kagan C Evans J Kay B 1986 A manual of interpersonal skills for nurses: an experiential approach. Harper & Row, London

Ley P 1988 Communicating with patients. Chapman and Hall, London

Mackereth P 1997 Clinical supervision for 'potent' practice. Complementary Therapies in Nursing and Midwifery 3 (2): 38–42

Mackereth P 1999 An introduction to catharsis and the healing crisis in reflexology. Complementary Therapies in Nursing and Midwifery 5: 69–74

Mitchell A Cormack M 1998 Complementary medicine: a practical guide. Butterworth Heinemann, Oxford

Nelson-Jones R 1986 The theory and practice of counselling psychology. Cassell, London

Orr J 1988 Social skills. In: Rankin-Box D (ed) Complementary health therapies: a guide for nurses and the caring professions. Chapman and Hall, London

Palmer S Dainow S Milner P (eds) 1996 Counselling: The BAC counselling reader. Sage, London

Reading A E 1981 Psychological preparations for surgery: patient recall of information. Journal of Psychosomatic Research 25: 57–62

Rogers C R 1961 On becoming a person. Houghton Mifflin, Boston

Rogers C R 1980 A way of being. Houghton Mifflin, Boston

Stewart I 1989 T A counselling in action. Sage, London

Stewart I 1996 Developing transactional analytical counselling. Sage, London

Stewart W 1992 An A–Z of counselling theory and practice. Chapman & Hall, London

Taub H A, Baker M I 1983 The effect of repeated testing upon comprehension of informed consent materials by elderly volunteers. Experimental Aging Research 9: 135–138

Truax C B Carkuff R R 1967 Towards effective counselling and psychotherapy. Aldine, Chicago

Tschudin V 1995 Counselling skills for nurses. Baillière Tindall, London

Van Ooijen E Charnock A 1994 Sexuality and patient care. Chapman & Hall, London

Wilkinson S 1991 Factors which influence how nurses communicate with cancer patients. Journal of Advanced Nursing 16: 677–688

USEFUL ADDRESSES

Listed below are organizations which either offer counselling training or are useful reference points for particular client groups. Some, such as Relate, cover both areas.

Alcoholics Anonymous
PO Box 1
Stonebow House
Stonebow
York YOI 2NJ

BACUP (British Association of
Cancer United Patients)
3 Bath Place
Rivington Street
London EC2A 3JR

British Association for Counselling
37a Sheep Street
Rugby
Warwickshire CV21 3BX

Centre for Counselling and
Psychotherapy Education
21 Lancaster Rd
London
WII 1QL

Childline
Freepost 1111
London W1H OBR

CRUSE
126 Sheen Rd
Richmond TW9 1UR

MIND
The White Building
Fitzalan Square
Sheffield S1 2AY

Relate
Herbert Gray College
Little Church Street
Rugby
Warwickshire CV21 3A

21 Healing

Denise Rankin-Box

Healing – the practice of conscious intentionality to improve health and well-being.

Healing may take many forms, such as faith healing, the 'laying on of hands' or ritual Shamanism, and is one of the oldest and most widespread forms of health care. Even today it is highly sought after, as reflected by the estimated number (over 20 000) of healers practising in the UK (Fulder & Monroe 1981, Turton 1988). Benor (1991) reported 8000 healers were registered in 16 different organizations in the UK and working under a unified code of conduct; these organizations also provide formal instruction in healing.

Alongside the reductionist approach of conventional medicine health care, religious or spiritual healing beliefs and practices seem to be flourishing (Glik 1990). There is also a growing body of literature on the origins of healing and healing belief systems (Easthope 1985, Benor 1990, Glik 1990, Graham 1999, see also Chapter 10, Sacred Space). Amongst the many terms used to refer to healing are 'faith', 'spiritual', 'psychic', 'paranormal' and 'shamanistic' (Benor 1990). The 'shaman – scientist' (Achterberg 1985, see also chapter 11, Shamanism) is attempting to link ancient intuitive practices and modern medicine. According to Graham (1999), Shamans were attributed with a range of powers including mastery of natural lore, healing the sick, telepathy and clairvoyance. They were also priests, mystics or poets. Perhaps new health care models will look to the original Hippocratic model of 2000 years ago which held that – 'there is one flow; one common breathing; all things are in sympathy' (Graham 1991).

There are many forms of healing and only those most commonly encountered can be described here. However, key issues addressing facets of healing have been addressed in more depth in Approaches to Healing, Section 2 of this book. These chapters have tried to exemplify the breadth of healing approaches and their potential within health care. Two features that these different practices have in common are:

- close links with a belief system which may be religious, spiritual, social or cultural
- the belief that healers channel healing 'energy' to the client.

A healing session usually involves assessment of the client's energy field and the passage of energy to them through the healer by gentle touch or a light sweeping of the healer's hands near the client's body. In addition, more complex rituals may be used. Healers may also treat by distant healing, using thought, intent, meditation or prayer to project healing to a client who may be some distance away (Benor 1991).

Healing has been performed safely in the clinical setting and particular forms seem to be effective for pain relief, relaxation and in promoting wound healing and reducing postoperative pain (Beutler et al 1988, Wirth et al 1993a, 1993b). Clearly, healing should not be performed without the client's consent and ideally the form used should be in accordance with their own beliefs.

HISTORICAL BACKGROUND

The sheer diversity of healing practices and the belief systems from which they arise makes it difficult to provide a general history. Archaeological and anthropological evidence suggests that healing is rooted in ancient shamanistic practices, linked to magic and mystery (Achterberg 1985, Graham 1986, 1991, 1999, see also chapter 11, Shamanism). Mystic tradition views the universe or cosmos as 'one'; everything is interrelated (including people). A mystic/healer may have an enhanced perception of this universe and, along with heightened sensitivity and awareness, uses certain rituals to interpret and work with the universal forces.

Shamanism is commonly attributed to the Tungus, Siberian tribes, but shamanistic methods seem to have been in use as far back as 20 000 years. Shaman healers were engaged in maintaining the harmony both of individuals and of the tribe. They were considered to have certain powers aligned with the natural forces of the environment. They had a knowledge of plants and herbs, were skilled in healing rituals and were able to communicate with the spirits. The shaman was an holistic practitioner, attempting to harmonize individual and environment (see chapter 11, Shamanism).

In ancient Greece, the life-force was perceived as being a state of dynamic harmony (Graham 1991). Any problems, such as illness, were due to disharmony affecting the life-force. Similarly, Egyptian medicine considered the condition of the whole person, although there were different healers for different problems. Hippocrates' approach to health care also focused on harmony. He emphasized nature's healing power – the vix medicatrix (Graham 1991) – and his students studied the effects of the seasons and the elements on health in a model not dissimilar to that of traditional Chinese medicine.

In the early fourteenth century, climatic changes resulted in crop failures and starvation across Europe. Together with unhygienic living conditions, this led to the spread of the disease Black Death which wiped out up to one half of Europe's population. The survival rate of women was seven times that of men and many believed that women were using some form of magic not only to survive but also to kill men (Achterberg 1990). The rise of Christianity in Europe directly influenced the practice of healing which was claimed as the exclusive domain of the church (Turton 1988). Women healers continued to function under the close eye of the church but, by the late 1300s, women were banned from officially training in medicine and it was claimed that they must have acquired their knowledge from the devil. The churches' position was 'that if a woman dare to cure without having studied, she is a witch and must die' (Michelet 1939). Any woman practising healing outside the auspices of the church was subject to extreme persecution and many were labelled witches and burnt at the stake (Turton 1988). As a result, any knowledge of healing practices of the time can only be deduced from records of witchcraft trials (Graham 1991, Rankin-Box 1999).

Despite these controls, the practice of healing continued. One notable healer was Valentine Greatrakes whose healing powers were in considerable demand in the 1700s (Harvey 1983, Turton 1988). Greatrakes was one of the first healers to invite scientific scrutiny of his work (Turton 1988). At this time, women were still being burnt at the stake for similar healing practices. The antagonism between church and lay healers continued and as recently as 1951 it was still theoretically possible to be arrested under the Witchcraft Act which held the death penalty (MacManaway & Turcan 1983).

TREATMENT

There are an increasing number of studies that demonstrate the positive effects of particular forms of healing, and indeed Benor (1990, see also chapter 14, Healing Research) when reviewing research on spiritual healing, commented that if healing were a drug it would be accepted as effective on the basis of current research results. Healing can be of benefit in a number of clinical settings. Benor (1990) reviewed 131 controlled trials of healing and concluded that 56 of these demonstrated a positive effect. A few of the many forms of healing are described next.

Lay healing – many healers claim to have no specific religious faith or beliefs influencing the healing process. There is usually some concept of rebalancing the client's energy or of the flow of energy between practitioner and client. A range of gentle techniques may be used during the healing experience and healing may also be conducted at a distance.

Spiritual healing – the laying on of hands or healing by prayer/meditation in which a special state of mind is required for healing to occur (Benor 1990). Spiritual healing is closely linked to a belief or faith system. The healer seeks to act as a channel for spiritual energy to flow through to the client. This may occur directly or from a distance.

Reiki – an interactive approach where healing energy is transferred from healer to client. The aim is to restore balance in the client's energy field (Wirth et al 1993a). A range of techniques may be used during healing, such as visualization and the laying on of hands.

LeShan – this technique is not based on an energy theory but advocates that the healer attains an enhanced state of consciousness in order for a 'flow process reality' to occur (Wirth et al 1993). LeShan believed that everyone has a natural ability for healing which can be accessed using the appropriate technique (LeShan 1974, Wirth et al 1993).

Shamanism – this generally refers to specific tribes engaged in maintaining the psychic and ecological equilibrium of their existence (Graham 1991). The shaman's healing powers rely on intuition and interpretation of images. They involve an enhanced state of consciousness induced by using stimulants, rhythmic swaying or other movement, meditation or chanting. Various forms have been described in Polynesia, China, Africa, South Pacific and the Americas (Graham 1991).

Stages of technique

Healing can occur in a special centre, at home or at a distance. A session may last from a few minutes to an hour and several sessions may be needed over a period of time. The client might be treated sitting or lying down. The stages of treatment are usually as follows:

Centring – initial preparation in which the healer becomes relaxed, calm and focused on the care about to be given.

Assessment – the healer may pass his/her hands quickly over the body or head, not usually touching the skin. Temperature changes may be identified by the healer, indicating imbalances of energy.

Healing – stroking or sweeping gestures may be used to balance the client's energy field. Conversely a holding technique may be used on or around the client's body in an attempt to direct energy. Prayers or words may be spoken.

Healing is generally a soothing, gentle experience and clients may experience tingling sensations or temperature changes.

Therapeutic potential in nursing

The possible applications of healing in nursing practice include:

- post-operative pain (dental) (Wirth et al 1993a)
- wound healing (Wirth et al 1990b)
- relaxation
- tension headaches
- anxiety
- hypertension.

Healing does not generally cure but it may initiate a positive process of

Contraindications for use

- There appear to be minimal side-effects; occasionally a sensation of light-headedness or faintness may occur.
- It is most important that the client is a willing participant, particularly for methods based on cultural and spiritual belief systems.

Summary

Healing is a gentle, non-invasive form of care that commonly instils feelings of relaxation and calmness (Vickers 1993). It does not require any equipment apart from the healer's hands, one of the key forms of communication at a nurse's disposal (Turton 1988). Healing offers a means of caring for clients in a personal way and may be particulaly suited to nursing practice.

REFERENCES

Achterberg J 1985 Imagery in healing. Shamanism and modern medicine. New Science Library, Boston
Achterberg J 1990 Woman as healer. Rider Random Century, London
Benor D J 1990 Survey of spiritual healing research. Complementary Medical Research 4: 9–33
Benor D J 1991 Spiritual healing in clinical practice. Nursing Times 87: 35–37
Beutler J, Attevelt J, Schouten S, Faber J, Mees E, Geuskes G 1988 Paranormal healing and hypertension. British Medical Journal 230: 1491–1494
Easthope G 1985 Three marginal healers. In: Jones K (ed) Sickness and sectarianism. Gower, London
Fulder S J, Monroe R 1981 The status of complementary medicine in the UK. Threshold Foundation

Glik D C 1990 The redefinition of the situation in the social construction of spiritual healing experiences. Sociology of Health and Illness 12: 151–168

Graham H 1986 The human face of psychology. Humanistic psychology in its historical, social and cultural context. Open University Press, Milton Keynes

Graham H 1991 The return of the Shaman: the emergence of a biophysical approach to health and healing. Complementary Medical Research 5(3): 165–171

Graham H 1999 Complementary therapies in context: the psychology of healing. Jessica Kinsley, London

Harvey D 1983 The power to heal. An investigation of healing and the healing experience. Aquarian Press, London

LeShan L 1974 The medium, the mystic and the physicist: towards a general theory of the paranormal. Viking Press, New York

MacManaway B, Turcan J 1983 Healing. Thorsons, Wellingborough

Michelet J 1939 Satanism and witchcraft. Translated by Allinson W R 1860 (Secaucas N J: Citadel 1939) Cited in Achterberg J 1990 Woman as healer. Rider Random Century, London

Rankin-Box D 1999 Paradoxes, puzzles and passing time. Complementary Therapies in Nursing and Midwifery 5 (6): 151–154

Turton P 1988 Healing: Therapeutic Touch. In: Rankin-Box D F (ed) Complementary health therapies: a guide for nurses and the caring professions. Croom Helm, Beckenham

Vickers A 1993 Complementary medicine and disability: alternatives for people with disabling conditions. Chapman and Hall, London

Wirth D P Brenlan D R Levine R J Rodriguez C M 1993a The effect of complementary healing therapy on postoperative pain after surgical removal of impacted third molar teeth. Complementary Therapies in Medicine 1: 133–138

Wirth D P Richardson J T Eidelman W C O'Malley A C 1993b Full thickness dermal wounds treated with non-contact therapeutic touch: a replication and extension. Complementary Therapies in Medicine 1: 127–132

USEFUL ADDRESSES

British Alliance of Healing
Associations
26 Highfield Avenue
Herne Bay
Kent CT6 6LM
Tel: 01227 3738 04

Confederation of Healing
Organisations
Suite J, 2nd Floor
The Red and White House
113 High Street
Berkhamstead
Hertfordshire HP4 2DJ
Tel: 01442 870661

Greater World Christian Spiritual
Association
3–5 Conway Street
Fitzrovia
London W1P 5HA
Tel: 020 7436 7555

National Federation of Spiritual
Healers
Old Manor Farm Studio
Sunbury-on-Thames Church
Middlesex TW16 6RG
Tel: 01932 783164
E-mail: office@NFSH.org.uk.

Sacred Space Foundation
Redmire
Mungrisdale
Cumbria CA11 0TB
Tel: 0176 877 9000
Fax: 0176 877 9111

Westbank Healing and Teaching
Centre
Strathmiglo
Fife
Scotland KY14 7QP

World Federation of Healing
6 Whitworth House
Buckhurst House
Bexhill-on-Sea
East Sussex TN40 1UA
Tel: 01424 214457

22 Herbal medicine

Helen Busby

Herbal medicine – *the use of whole plant material by trained practitioners to promote recovery from disease and to enable healing to take place.*

Herbalists treat a wide range of conditions, similar to those with which people present to their General Practitioners. Patients of all ages, including infants and pregnant women, can be safely treated with herbs by a qualified experienced practitioner.

Many people use herbal medicine as a treatment of choice (Sharma 1992). Older people, in particular, may continue a long-held allegiance to herbal remedies, and an increasing number of parents see herbal medicine as a gentle first recourse for their children. However, many people turn to a herbalist only after conventional approaches have proved less than satisfactory for their particular condition. This may still be beneficial since herbal treatment is particularly valuable in promoting recovery from various complex conditions.

In an international context, the World Health Organization has recognized the considerable importance of herbal medicine to meeting health needs (WHO 1978). In the UK, the role of the professional herbalist was recognized in the 1968 Medicines Act, which makes provision for particularly potent herbal medicines that are not permitted for over-the-counter sale to be prescribed by a professional herbalist. The National Institute of Medical Herbalists (NIMH), founded in 1864, now oversees standards of practice and ensures high standards of training.

Herbal medicine is at present little used within nursing in the UK, with the exception of the external use of essential oils from herbs for massage (aromatherapy). In European countries such as France and Germany, where herbal medicine is more integrated into the health care system, it is usually the physician who has the responsibility for prescribing the herbs. It is suggested then, that it is the traditional divisions of labour and roles between nurses and physicians, rather than any lack of therapeutic potential, which are primarily responsible for the limited use of herbal medicine within nursing. This challenge to conventional roles will need to be addressed before the therapeutic potential of herbal medicine is likely to be fulfilled. There are a number of small projects, particularly in the area of drug and alcohol dependence, where nurses with additional specialized training in herbal medicine are able to use these skills with their patients.

The practice of herbal medicine requires substantial training (currently 4 years full-time or equivalent part-time) and the therapy is, in the British Medical Association's words, a 'discrete clinical entity' (BMA 1993) rather than a set of techniques.

HISTORICAL BACKGROUND

Herbal medicine has been at the core of most systems of medicine throughout history. Historical sources, including herbals, provide us with information about traditions and systems of herbal medicines from at least the first century BC in ancient Greek, Egyptian and Chinese cultures. However, mythologies suggest, and archaeological findings confirm, that use of herbal medicine began many thousands of years earlier (Griggs 1981). An account by Theophrastus of the medicinal uses of 455 plants, written in the third century BC, was probably the earliest Western herbal. The advent of printing in the sixteenth and seventeenth centuries made it possible for herbals like Culpeper's, published in 1652, to have a wide circulation.

Today, about a quarter of pharmaceutical preparations contain at least one active constituent extracted from plant sources (Farnsworth 1981). Well-known examples among the thousands of drugs originally discovered from plants include digitalis (from Foxglove), aspirin (from Willow and Meadowsweet) and ephedrine (from the Chinese Ephedra).

TREATMENT

A key to herbal treatment is the emphasis on the 'vital force' or life energy of the patient, and mobilizing the self-healing or homeostatic powers of the body. One implication of this is that the patient's subjective experience of their symptoms is central to the diagnostic process. A detailed case history will be taken as part of the initial consultation, including information that will help the herbalist to assess the personal and social context of an individual's illness or disease. A Western herbalist will use a similar system of diagnosis to current orthodox medicine, with particular emphasis on aetiology.

A herbalist will choose from plants which have general actions, including relaxant, tonic, enhancement of immune resistance, or more specific actions, such as vasodilatory, hypotensive, anti-inflammatory, expectorant and diuretic (Weiss 1988). Different constituents of a prescription or within a single plant combine to form a total effect which is 'more than the sum of the parts', known as synergy. For example, the anti-inflammatory action of the aspirin-like salicylates in Meadowsweet is buffered by a range of other constituents which soothe and protect the mucosa of the digestive tract, making use of the total plant material safer than its chemical counterpart.

Herbs are prescribed in a number of forms:

- infusions (herb teas)
- decoctions (roots or barks simmered in water)
- tinctures (concentrated extracts of a herb in a solution of water and alcohol)
- juices
- capsules
- external applications, such as creams, lotions or poultices.

The length of treatment varies according to individual need, but as with many therapies, chronic problems generally take several months, whilst acute problems, even if more severe, are likely to respond in a matter of days or weeks.

Therapeutic potential

Herbal medicine can be effective for a wide range of health problems. Some examples are:

- Vasodilatory (Weiss 1988)
- Cardiovascular system (Ernest 1987)
- Migraines (Murphy et al 1988)
- Anti-inflammatory (Weiss 1988)
- Skin conditions (Sheehan et al 1992)

Contraindications for use

There are few absolute contraindications for the use of herbal medicine by trained practitioners. Contrary to popular belief, not all herbs are safe in all situations. For example:

- Liquorice is not recommended for long-term use by people with hypertension
- Ginseng should not be taken by a person with significant levels of anxiety, tension or restlessness or when there is acute inflammation.

Some conditions associated with organic damage are unlikely to respond to treatment with herbal medicine:

- Certain specific conditions, for example epilepsy, cannot be effectively treated with herbs

Contraindications for use (Cont'd)

- In some cases, such as severe mental illness or distress, herbal treatment could be supportive only in conjunction with appropriate support from a mental health team.

In some conditions, another therapy will be the treatment of choice. For example, insulin-dependent diabetes is best managed by an orthodox physician and some musculoskeletal conditions should be referred for treatment by an osteopath.

Interactions between herbal medicines and other prescribed medicines are possible, for example:

- The trained herbalist would avoid the use of Ephedra with monoamine oxidase inhibitors (MAOIs)
- Some herbs containing cardioactive glycosides, such as Lily of the Valley, would not be prescribed in conjunction with digitalis as they could potentiate each other.

Appropriate use and dosage of herbs, prescribed by trained herbalists, is the key to safety.

Summary

Herbal medicine has a wide range of applications within health care and has a well established historic ancestry. It can be a gentle and highly effective system of health care. Although herbal medicine is currently little used in nursing practice, nurses should be familiar with its use and if giving advice to patients, should ensure they are competent to do so. Herbal medicine should only be prescribed by trained herbalists.

REFERENCES

BMA 1993 Complementary medicines: new approaches to good practice. British Medical Association/Oxford University Press, Oxford
Ernest E 1987 Cardiovascular effects of garlic: a review. Pharmathopeutica 5: 83–89
Farnsworth N 1981 Foreword to Griggs B Green pharmacy: a history of herbal medicine. Jill Norman and Hobhouse, London
Griggs B 1981 Green pharmacy: a history of herbal medicine. Jill Norman and Hobhouse, London
Murphy J J et al 1988 Randomised double-blind placebo-controlled trial of Feverfew in migraine prevention. Lancet ii: 189–192
Sharma U 1992 Complementary medicine today: practitioners and patients. Tavistock/Routledge, London (Chapter 1 contains an overview of some recent surveys of the extent of use of specified complementary medicines)

Sheehan M P et al 1992 Efficacy of traditional Chinese herbal therapy in adult atopic dermatitis. Lancet 340: 13–17

Weiss R F (trans. by Meuss A R) 1988 Herbal medicine. Beaconsfield, Beaconsfield

WHO 1978 The promotion and development of traditional medicine. World Health Organization (WHO) technical report series No. 662. WHO, Geneva

FURTHER READING – JOURNALS

The following journals will be useful for reviewing current practice and research:

The European Journal of Herbal Medicine

The Journal of Phytotherapy

Herbalgram

Greenfiles, a quarterly newsletter of research abstracts primarily for holistic practitioners is available from 'Greenfiles' at:

138 Oak Tree Lane

Mansfield

Notts N18 3HR

FURTHER READING – BOOKS

Fulder S 1990 The Tao of medicine: Ginseng and other Chinese herbs for inner equilibrium and immune power. Healing Arts Press, Vermont

Hoffman D 1990 The new holistic herbal. Element Books, Dorset

McIntyre A 1988 Herbs in pregnancy and childbirth. Sheldon Press, London

Weiss R F 1988 (trans. by Meuss, A R) Herbal medicine. Beaconsfield Publishers, London

OTHER RESOURCES

The following websites, together with the links they contain, will be useful for updating current research and policy:

National Institute of Medical Herbalists –
http://www.btinternet.com/~nimh/

The European Herbal Practitioners Association –
http://www.users.globalnet.co.uk/~ehpa/

Medicines Control Agency – http://open.gov.uk/mca/mlx249.htm

European Medicines Evaluation Agency – http://www.eudra.org/emea.html

TRAINING

The National Institute of Medical Herbalists can provide a list of qualified practitioners and a list of courses, including several degree courses, in herbal medicine.

National Institute of Medical Herbalists
56 Longbrook Street,
Exeter
Devon EX4 6AH
Tel: 01392 426022

23 Homeopathy

Kenneth Atherton

Homeopathy – *a 200-year-old system of medicine (Haehl 1985) based on the Law of Similars (let like be cured by like). The principle of homeopathy can be illustrated as follows: within seconds of being stung by the common garden nettle, a red, blotchy and often itchy rash appears. Yet the same nettle can be used to produce a homeopathic remedy which may stimulate the body's own capacity to heal itself by producing an opposite curative effect. Also, shell fish allergies or generalized urticaria may well respond to a homeopathic medicine made from the nettle, because although the causes differ the characteristics of the complaint are 'similar'.*

Homeopathic medicines or remedies are produced from various natural sources – plants, metals, minerals, venoms and stings, and also bacteria or human tissue; for example, extracts of the plant Belladonna (Deadly Nightshade), calcium carbonate (a layer of the oyster shell), lachesis (the venom of the deadly Bushmaster Snake) and bacteria such as *Pneumococcus* (Boericke 1987).

Effectivity results from the process by which remedies are made. The original substances are normally diluted many times in a water and alcohol base. At each dilution, the mixture is shaken vigorously, a process known as 'succussion', which homeopaths believe gives the final product its power to heal (Livingston 1991). Recent research by the French scientist Jacques Benveniste of the South Paris University suggests that the water/alcohol solution retains the memory of its original substance. Benveniste (1988) reported degranulation of basophils and histamine release when exposed to anti-IgE antibodies at dilutions that were so great that not one single molecule of anti-IgE was present (Benveniste 1988). Dr David Taylor-Reilly of the Glasgow Homeopathic Hospital compares this phenomenon to the ability of water to form many thousands of variations of snowflake shape. It is suggested that this 'memory' could be the underlying mechanism of homeopathy (Benveniste 1988).

Potencies are obtained according to accepted pharmaceutical principles. There are two forms of dilution, decimal and centesimal,

Table 23.1 *Table title*

Dilution	Concentration		Decimal scale	Centesimal scale
1/10	10%	10^{-1}	D1 or 1×	
1/100	1%	10^{-2}	D2 or 2×	1c or 1cH 1/100
1/1000	0.1%	10^{-3}	D3 or 3×	
1/10000	0.01%	10^{-4}	D4 or 4×	2c or 2cH 1/10000
1/100000	0.001%	10^{-5}	D5 or 5×	
1/1000000	0.0001%	10^{-6}	D6 or 6×	3c or 3cH 1/1000000
1/10		10^{-12}	D12 or 12×	6c or 6cH 1/10
		10^{-18}		9c 1/10
		10^{-24}		12c 1/10
		10^{-60}		30c 1/10
				200c
				1000c or 1M

successive methods of reduction being in steps of 1/10 and 1/100 respectively. The number of stages determines the potency of the dilution or trituration obtained as shown in the table above.

Homeopathic medicines are dispensed in four forms depending on the type of prescription:

- powders
- granules
- tablets
- liquids.

The following two examples illustrate prescribing techniques. In the case of powders, it is usual only to medicate the first two or three and follow with a series of unmedicated ones. The reason for this is to allow the medicated part of the prescription time to act. The therapeutic response varies in patients and may take several days to several weeks. Generally this type of prescription is written as follows:

Arsen Alb 1M 1–3   Arsen alb 30 in powders 1 to 3
S.L.12 t.d.s., p.c.   Lactose powders 4 to 12
                     One powder to be taken dry on the tongue three times a day after meals in the order numbered; 4 days' supply

Prescribing habits differ and sometimes a low potency may be given over a course of weeks or months. In these cases, tablets are often used. The tablets are composed of lactose with an added amount of pure sugar. The desired potency of the homeopathic medicine is absorbed into each tablet. An example of a prescription for tablets is as follows:

Gelsemium 6 c 7 g (50 tablets)
1 t.d.s.

Most pharmacies instruct patients undertaking homeopathic treatment to avoid coffee, peppermint or menthol, as these substances are considered to counteract the effect of the remedies. Homeopathic medicines in low potencies are readily available over the counter and it is commonplace now to see such preparations in pharmacies and health food shops. These medicines are generally available to the public for self-treatment; for example, Rhus Tox 6c for rheumatism or Chammomilla 6c for teething problems. However, for complex or chronic conditions, a skilled assessment and prescription is often necessary for which a qualified practitioner should be consulted.

Critics have for many years attributed successful homeopathic treatment to the 'placebo' effect. However, the growing amount of animal research would suggest otherwise. Veterinary surgeon, Christopher Day, carried out a double-blind trial in 1988 on mastitis in cows. The cows were split into two groups and treated over a 12-month period. Group A received a placebo in the form of untreated liquid drops added to the drinking water while for Group B liquid drops containing a homeopathic medicine were used. The results showed that the cows treated by homeopathy substantially improved and had fewer relapses than those given the placebo (Day 1988).

Homeopathy is complementary to conventional medicine, and may be particularly helpful in the alleviation of chronic ailments without the risk of side effects (Koehler 1986).

Training

The Faculty of Homeopathy at The Royal London Hospital, Great Ormond Street, London is the only statutory recognized training body (Act of Parliament, 1950) and its Academic Department offers the postgraduate qualifications LFHom, VetMFHom, DDFHom to doctors, dentists, veterinary surgeons, pharmacists, midwives and registered nurses.

Many lay people, however, still embark on self-funded courses set up by various independent homeopathic organizations throughout the UK. None of these courses offer a statutory recognized qualification as yet, therefore their students eventually practise under Common Law. In the future this type of training may have to alter under European Directives (Collins/Lannoye 1994). It has been suggested that lay homeopaths without a medical background or practical hospital experience might be less likely to know when to refer a patient for conventional medical opinion (Faculty of Homeopathy 1993).

However, recently two British universities have accredited BSc degrees in Homeopathy which can be undertaken by anybody with the appropriate university entrance requirements. One of the universities has included some conventional medical training as part of its programme; this may be an advantage should legislation to practise alter within the UK.

HISTORICAL BACKGROUND

The dominant name in the history of homeopathy is that of Hahnemann. The son of a porcelain painter of the Meissen factory in Saxony, Samuel Hahnemann (1755–1843) was a skilled linguist and translator before becoming a chemist and later a physician at the age of 24. It was while translating the Materia Medica of Professor Cullen of Edinburgh that Hahnemann realized the significance of homeopathic principles.

Hahnemann's first experiments involved the effects of quinine (Chinchona bark), reputed to cure malaria. The resemblance between the effects of quinine and the effects of malaria itself seemed to him more than coincidence (Livingston 1991). Hahnemann self-prescribed repeated doses of pure quinine and developed symptoms similar to those of malaria. He found that dilutions of the drug prepared in a homeopathic way were effective in curing malaria. Subsequently, many substances were tested on healthy volunteers to determine the symptoms they could produce and so cure. This form of experimentation is known as a 'proving'. Hahnemann's methods and teachings were not without their critics but his reputation spread widely. When towards the end of his life he moved to Paris, people waited in their carriages for days in order to consult him.

A post-graduate school of homeopathy was established late in the nineteenth century in Philadelphia, USA (Tyler-Kent 1979). Homeopathic hospitals developed in various major cities throughout the UK, including London, Liverpool, Glasgow, Bristol and Tunbridge Wells. Many of these hospitals still exist and are fully recognized under the NHS, patients being referred in the usual way through their GP. All these hospitals are staffed by qualified medical doctors who have undertaken further post-graduate training in homeopathic medicine.

TREATMENT

No condition, no matter how serious or trivial, is beyond homeopathic consideration. In advanced stages of terminal illness, substantial pain relief and comfort may be attained. The homeopathic approach to treatment differs from the conventional. Hahnemann was explicit about how a case history should be recorded and warned against the practitioner being biased or not allowing patients time to describe their symptoms (Koehler 1986). Every symptom is noted as described by the patient, accompanied by the practitioner's observations. Factors possibly considered of little importance conventionally can in homeopathy be crucial in the choice of a remedy. For example, although two people may present with a similar painful joint, one may report it worse during mobility and the other worse for rest; each would receive a completely different remedy. The choice of any remedy is always based on the totality of the symptoms (Livingston 1991).

A homeopath will often enquire about the patient's preferences, such as whether they feel more comfortable in a hot or cold environment, whether they have a desire or aversion for sweet foods, salt, condiments, fruit, eggs, fat, cheese or meat. All this information influences the choice of the correct remedy (Agrawal 1980). Questions about general health, sleep, bowel habits, childhood illnesses, alcohol and tobacco intake, family history and, most importantly, the patient's psychological condition will all contribute to the final decision regarding treatment (Boyd 1981). Routine investigations such as temperature, pulse, respiration, blood pressure, weight and laboratory tests are performed as necessary.

Therapeutic potential in nursing

Nurses trained in homeopathy as a first aid could contribute a great deal to nursing practice. Homeopathy has much to offer in community care, day nursing, industry, midwifery and nursing homes. It would also be useful in Accident and Emergency Departments, intensive care and medical and surgical units, provided the appropriate authorization is obtained.

Some acute complaints that can be treated are as follows:

- Accident and emergency:
  sudden collapse – Carbo Veg
  acute injuries – Arnica
  Injured nerves – Hypericum
- Bites and stings:
  wasps or bees – Apis Mel, Urtica Urens, Ledum
- Burns and scalds:
  severe blistering – Cantharis
  sunburn – Belladonna
  local application – Calendula
- Care of the chronically and terminally ill, including pain management and emotional distress:
  terminal illness with restlessness – Arsen Alb
  pains associated with tumours – Euphorbium
  distressed relatives – Gelsemium, Ignatia
- Chemotherapy and radiotherapy – to assist with nausea and general health:
  skin tenderness after radiotherapy – Cantharis

Therapeutic potential in nursing (Cont'd)

- Community care – with a wide application for district nursing in the treatment of wounds and leg ulcers and care of the elderly: postoperative wounds – Arnica, Staphysagria leg ulcers – Calendula, Flouric Acid

- Coughs, colds, sore throats and influenza: influenza – Gelsemium, Aconite fever – Belladonna coughs – Bryonia

- Distressed relatives, e.g. shock and grief reactions: shock – Gelsemium, Aconite grief – Ignatia

- Endoscopic procedures: pre-general anaesthetic – Phosphorus apprehensive patients – Gelsemium, Argentum Nitrate

- First aid – road traffic accidents, including air, sea and mountain rescue (as for accident and emergency)

- Hayfever and simple allergies – Homeopathic Grass Pollen, Allium Cepa

- Hyperactive children – Belladonna, Agaricus

- Insomnia – Coffea

- Midwifery (pre- and post-natal care): miscarriage prevention – Caulophyllum injuries associated with childbirth – Arnica, Staphysagria

- Pre- and post-surgical management including dental surgery: before any surgical procedure – Arnica

- Stress and phobias – including anticipation and fear of unpleasant investigations and surgical procedures phobic states – Phosphorus, Argentum Nitrate anticipatory fear – Gelsemium.

Contraindications for use

On the whole, homeopathic treatment is safe and will not interfere with conventional medicines prescribed by the patient's GP. However, some homeopaths feel that treatment may be less effective if combined with drugs, particularly steroid preparations.

Contraindications are few but the following categories are important:

- Patients known to have sensitivity to milk products should inform their homeopath as lactose is often used as a tablet base for the homeopathic remedy. Remedies can then be supplied in a water and alcohol base in the form of drops.

- Diabetic patients should inform the homeopath of their condition because of the lactose based medication. An alternative non-sugar based medication can be used.

- Young babies may not be able to metabolize alcohol, so remedies should be alcohol free. Alcohol-free medicine may be dissolved in a little water and administered via the feeding bottle.
- Where possible homeopaths should collaborate with medical colleagues and never attempt to treat a patient with a serious illness

Summary

Homeopathy can be surprisingly effective but patients must be prepared to give the treatment time to achieve a therapeutic response. This sometimes means a change in lifestyle, which could include an alteration in diet, more relaxation and exercise to complement the treatment.

REFERENCES

Agrawal V R 1980 A repertory of desires and aversions. Vijay, Delhi

Benveniste J 1988 Human basophil degranulation triggered by very dilute anti serum against IgE. Nature 333: 816–818

Boericke W 1987 Homoeopathic materia medica with repertory. Homoeopathic Book Service, London

Boyd H 1981 Introduction to homoeopathic medicine. Beaconsfield, Beaconsfield

Collins Lannoye P 1994 Report of the status of complementary medicine, Committee on the environment public health and consumer protection

Day C 1988 Clinical trials in bovine mastitis. British Homoeopathic Journal 75: 11–14

Faculty of Homoeopathy 1993 Non-medically qualified practitioners of homeopathy. British Homoeopathic Journal with Simile 82

Haehl R 1985 Samuel Hahnemann. His life and work. B Jain, New Delhi, India, 2 vols

Koehler G 1986 Handbook of homoeopathy. Thorsons, London

Livingston R 1991 Homoeopathy evergreen medicine. Jewel in the medical crown. Asher Asher, Poole

Tyler-Kent J 1979 Lectures in homoeopathic philosophy. Thorsons, Wellingborough

FURTHER READING – JOURNALS

Engineer S J Vakil A E Engineer L S 1990 A study of antibody formation by Baptisia tinctoria O in experimental animals. British Homoeopathic Journal 79: 109–113

Fox A D 1993 General practice management of gastrointestinal problems assisted by Vegatest techniques. British Homoeopathic Journal 82: 87–91

Gaucher C Jeulin D Peycru P Pla A Amengual C 1993 Cholera and homoeopathic medicine. British Homoeopathic Journal 82: 155–163

Jacobs J Jiminez L M Gloyd S Caraes F E Gaitan M P Crowthers D 1993 Homoeopathic treatment of acute childhood diarrhoea. British Homoeopathic Journal 82: 83–86

Linde W Melchart D Jonas W B Hornung J 1994 Ways to enhance the quality and acceptance of clinical and laboratory studies in homoeopathy. British Homoeopathic Journal 83: 3–7

Mokkapatti R 1992 An experimental double-blind study to evaluate the use of Euphrasia in preventing conjunctivitis. British Homoeopathic Journal 81: 22–24

Rastogi D P Singh V P Singh V Dey S K 1993 Evaluation of homoeopathic therapy in 129 asymptomatic HIV carriers. British Homoeopathic Journal 82: 4–8

Vozianov A F Simeonova N K 1990 Homoeopathic treatment of patients with adenomas of the prostate. British Homoeopathic Journal 79: 148–151

FURTHER READING – BOOKS

Blackie M 1986 Classical homoeopathy. Beaconsfield, Beaconsfield

Boyd H 1981 Introduction to homoeopathic medicine. Beaconsfield, Beaconsfield

Hubbard E W 1990 Homoeopathy as art and science. Beaconsfield, Beaconsfield

Livingston R 1991 Homeopathy evergreen medicine. Jewel in the medical crown. Asher Asher, Poole

Lockie A 1989 The family guide to homoeopathy. Hamish Hamilton, London

Resch G Gutmann V 1987 Scientific foundations of homoeopathy. Barthel and Barthel, St Ottillien, Germany

Smith T 1986 Talking about homoeopathy. Insight, Worthing

Tyler-Kent J 1979 Lectures in homoeopathic philosophy. Thorsons, Wellingborough.

USEFUL ADDRESSES

Any professional nurse interested in training in homeopathy should ensure that the course is nationally accredited and has statutory recognition. It is helpful to obtain a copy of the Faculty of Homoeopathy Statement entitled 'Non-medically qualified practitioners of homoeopathy' referred to in the Reference list.

Faculty of Homoeopathy
Academic Department
The Glasgow Homoeopathic
Hospital
1053 Great Western Road
Glasgow G42 OXQ
Tel: 0141 211 1616

Fax: 0141 211 1610
E-mail: info@trusthomeopathy.org
Website:
www.trusthomeopathy.org/faculty

Faculty of Homoeopathy
15 Clerkenwell Close
London EC1R 0AA
Tel: 020 7566 7810

Fax: 020 7566 7815
E-mail: info@trusthomeopathy.org
Website:
www.trusthomeopathy.org/faculty

*Faculty of Homeopathy Primary Health Care Examination (LFHom) qualification
for registered nurses and midwives.*
*Further advanced intermediate training for nurses in preparation.

Institute of Complementary
Medicine
PO Box 194
London SE16 1QZ
Tel: 020 7237 5165
Fax: 020 7237 5175
E-mail: icm@icmedicine.co.uk
Website: www.icmedicine.co.uk

Information available on degree
courses and NVQs in
complementary medicine.

Centre for the Study of
Complementary Medicine
(C.S.C.M.)
51 Bedford Place
Southampton
Hampshire SO1 2DG
Tel: 01703 334752
Fax: 01703 231835

E-mail:
cscm.compmed@btinternet.com
Website: www.complemed.co.uk.

Administration & Marketing Office
University of Westminster
115 New Cavendish Street
London W1M 8JG
Tel: 020 7911 5833
Fax: 020 7911 5079
E-mail: cavadmin@wmin.ac.uk
Website: www.wmin.ac.uk

Business Development Unit
University of Central Lancashire
Preston PR1 2HE
Tel: 01772 893835
Fax: 01772 892998
E-mail: (see Website)
Website: www.aclan.ac.uk

*The Centre offers post-graduate courses in the scientific evaluation of homoeopathic
therapy to medical doctors, dentists and registered nurses. Applicants should have a
background in homoeopathic medicine. The Centre has carried out much of the
leading scientific research in homoeopathic and complementary therapies and
publishes its findings on a regular basis.*

Humour and laughter therapy

Jane Mallett

Humour therapy – *a humorous intervention used by the health care professional or patient to produce a beneficial response in the patient.*
Laughter therapy – *an intervention used by the health care professional or patient to produce beneficial laughter in the patient.*

'Humour and laughter therapy and their effects are not necessarily mutually exclusive. However, humour can occur without laughter and laughter without humour.' Sultanoff (1994)

Humour can be viewed from physical, psychological and sociological perspectives and has been defined in a number of ways. Humour is reported to consist of wit (a thought-oriented experience), mirth (an emotionally-oriented experience) and laughter (a physiologically-oriented experience) (Sultanoff 1994). Laughter is generally taken to be the physical expression of humour (Keith-Spiegel 1972) although this does not take account of its use as a managed and organized conversational activity in its own right (see below) (Jefferson 1984, Jefferson et al 1987).

The physical responses to humour and laughter affect most of the major systems of the body (Fry 1986, Dunn 1993). These include an increase in heart rate, blood pressure and muscle tension which is followed by a decrease (Berlyne 1972, Chapman 1976, Fry 1986, Fry & Savin 1988, Dunn 1993). In addition, salivary immunoglobulin A (IgA) concentration and spontaneous lymphocyte blastogenesis have been found to increase, and adrenalin and cortisol secretion to decrease, following viewing of a humorous video by healthy adults (Dillon et al, 1985, Berk et al 1988a, 1988b). The clinical significance of this research is unclear but *may* turn out to have important implications for health care. However, authors have rightly questioned whether there is sufficient 'research' to support the conclusion that humour and laughter promote health and wellness (Sultanoff 1999).

Psychological research has shown that humour can have a part in reducing anxiety. A study by Nemeth (1979) indicated that people who watched a humorous film had significantly decreased anxiety levels compared with those who watched a non-humorous film. Sick joke cycles (e.g. following the Chernobyl disaster – 'What has feathers and glows in the dark?' 'Chicken Kiev') have been studied from a socio-logical perspective (Dundes 1987). It is suggested that these act as a collective mental defence mechanism to allow people to articulate and cope with the worst disasters (Dundes 1987). A survey of young Finnish families has also indicated that members use humour as a coping strategy when there are difficulties, such as disagreement, within the family (Åstedt-Kurki et al 1999).

In addition, there are cultural, sex and age differences in the use of humour and laughter. For instance, Eskimos have been reported to use humour to resolve quarrels – whoever gains most laughter from the audience while insulting their opponents wins the argument (Robinson 1977) – and differences have been found in the amount of laughter and smiling between males and females of different ages in a restaurant. Overall, females laughed and smiled more than males, with females aged 12–17 laughing most (Adams & Kirkevold 1978). This highlights that cultural, gender and age differences need to be taken into account when considering the use of humour and laughter as tools for therapy.

Importantly, humour and laughter are produced and responded to within context (Jefferson et al 1987, Norrick 1993, 1994) and enable a number of conversational activities – such as 'speaking off the record', reframing the current activity as 'play', negotiating topic changes and realignments etc (Norrick 1993, 1994). Humour and laughter can also lead to the development of affiliation and rapport (Jefferson et al 1987, Norrick 1993, 1994). Therefore, humour and laughter are more than talk or gestures merely intended to cause amusement but are utilized by participants in conversation to provide for a variety of outcomes.

The use of humour and laughter in health care situations between patients (Coser 1959), and health care professionals and patients (Emerson 1963, Ragan 1990, Mallett & A'Hern 1996, Mallett 1997) has also been explored. There is evidence that humour is used in a variety of health care situations including intensive care (Coombs & Goldman 1972), wards (Coser 1959, Emerson 1963, Savage 1992), child health and oncology clinics (Warner 1984, Inman 1988), gynaecological health clinics (Ragan 1990) and renal units (Mallett 1997).

Humour has been found to be integral to some nurse–patient conversations. Analysis of verbal and non-verbal video data of nurses teaching patients to haemodialyse indicated that out of 126 haemo-dialysis sessions of five patients 'humorous instances' were found in virtually all recordings (125) (Mallett & A'Hern 1996). The rate at which humour was produced and the proportion of humour constructed by patients in 'teaching sessions' were differentially distributed between patients. In addition, for one patient a significant positive relationship between the rate of humour per session and time was demonstrated and another was found to produce a significantly larger proportion of the humour over time. Further exploration revealed that in the latter case this *may* have been associated with the patient's anxiety and difficulties with regard to needling (Mallett & A'Hern 1996).

Research also indicates that humour and laughter is used contextually and spontaneously by nurses and patients to accomplish a number of outcomes including to:

- protest
- express fears
- raise issues
- send unofficial messages relating to death
- facilitate social interaction
- veil antagonism
- comment on staff competence
- overcome the face-threat of examination
- gain and maintain patient involvement
- highlight anxieties and difficulties
- demonstrate 'trouble-resistance'
- avoid conflict
- develop rapport
- disrupt thematic orientation during teaching (Emerson 1963, Ragan 1990, Mallett & A'Hern 1996, Mallett 1997).

In addition, there is some evidence from patients' and carers' stories and text that humour is used to cope with cancer (for example see Bruning 1985, Treadwell 1998, Saltman 1999a). For example, Bruning (1985), who discovered that she had breast cancer at the age of 31 and underwent chemotherapy, wrote how she sometimes 'spent more time joking and laughing than being treated'. Saltman's website, 'Kcuf recnac' (saltman 1999a), also ably illustrates the use of humour. Saltman refers to his diagnosis:

> 'The infectious disease specialist could come to no conclusions in her office and scheduled me for a biopsy to remove one of the lumps. This was done on Friday, 7 (8th?) March in a doctor's office. He simply novacained around the most prominent lump and swish swish with his knife took it out. It was about the size of a fingernail and looked a bit like cauliflower, but smoother. The surgeon wasn't too good-looking either.'   (Saltman 1999b)

Other beneficial effects are also demonstrated in patients' accounts. Cousins (1976), who suffered from ankylosing spondylitis, watched

Candid Camera films and found that 10 minutes of genuine belly laughter had an anaesthetic effect that would give him 2 hours of pain-free sleep.

Research of professionals' and patients' views demonstrates that both nurses and patients believe that humour and laughter have useful effects and/or are important to the nurse–patient relationship (Schmitt, 1990, Åstedt-Kurki & Liukkonen 1994, Fosbinder 1994). For instance, patients view nurses who laugh with them as therapeutic (Schmitt 1990) and nurses believe that humour can make the patients feel better in many ways (Åstedt-Kurki & Liukkonen 1994). Again there is also anecdotal evidence to support the use of humour in health care (Wooten 1999a).

The actual and potential effects of humour and laughter and how they are utilized within conversation have implications for the development of therapies in health care. This includes: the potential for ameliorating symptoms – for example, pain (Cousins 1976); the ability to facilitate communication by the management of interactional difficulties between nurses and patients and developing rapport (Mallett 1997); and the potential for enabling the patient to cope with their situation (Bruning 1985). However, while the value of humour is recognized by patients, humour may not always be appropriate (Goldklang 1996, Love 1998).

HISTORICAL BACKGROUND

The benefits of humour and laughter have long been recognized and are mentioned in the Bible; Proverbs 17:22 states 'A cheerful heart does good like a medicine: but a broken spirit makes one sick' (Living Bible 1971). More recently it has been suggested that humour and/or laughter may be used therapeutically in a number of ways (Moody 1978, Goldstein 1982):

- to aid recovery from surgery (Henri de Mondeville, thirteenth-century surgeon)
- as a cure for melancholy (Robert Burton, sixteenth-century English parson and scholar)
- as physical exercise (Richard Mulcaster, sixteenth-century physician)
- as a way to release excess tension (Herbert Spencer, seventeenth-century sociologist)
- to restore equilibrium (Immanuel Kant, eighteenth-century German philosopher)
- to use in treatment of the sick (William Battie, eighteenth-century English physician)

- to help digestion (Gottlieb Hufeland, nineteenth-century German professor)
- to stimulate the internal organs (James Walsh, twentieth-century American physician).

One of the most influential proponents of humour and laughter therapy of modern times who has probably been responsible for the upsurge in interest since the 1970s, is Norman Cousins. His documented experiences as a patient and subsequent writings on the value of humour and laughter in health care (Cousins 1976, 1979, 1989) have done much to stimulate the imagination of professionals. In addition, for the last 25 years Dr Hunter 'Patch' Adams has been one of America's leading proponents of humour in medicine (Burkeman 1998). Particularly in the USA, these types of therapies are currently popular and seem to have encouraged much supportive business (for example, the Humor Project).

TREATMENT

Humour or laughter therapy may take the form of making funny pictures to decorate the patient's room, sending singing telegrams, showing home or humorous movies, using puppets to increase playfulness and clowns to facilitate communication and responsiveness (Cousins 1976, Moody 1978, Simon 1989, Erdman 1991, Wooten 1999b, 1999c).

Literature describing humour or laughter therapy in clinical practice is sparse, although Erdman (1991) and Wooten (1999a) highlight the use of a 'Laugh Mobile' and 'Humour Cart'. The 'Laugh Mobile' was wheeled round to patients in their rooms twice a week. Examples of items on the Laugh Mobile included: Play Doh (a soft modelling clay), colouring books, finger paint, Mr Bubble® (a pipe for blowing bubbles), water guns, humorous books, videotapes and audiotapes, games and puzzles. Erdman (1991) describes the 'success' of the therapy and illustrates this with examples of how patients reacted:

> 'A 42-year-old patient with lymphoma was the first patient to select Mr Bubble from the humour cart. He laughed like a child as he blew sparkly bubbles that burst when they touched his smiling visitors.' (p. 1362)

The Humour Cart, developed by Terry Bennett for cancer patients in Philadelphia, is left in the hospital hallway so people can view the contents. It includes videos, comedy audiotapes, toys – such as squirt guns, Mr Potato Head, yo yo's, kaleidoscopes – funny costumes, polaroid camera, etc. The most popular video is by Joe Kogel, a cancer survivor, called 'Life and Death' (Wooten 1999a).

Humour as a means of facilitating communication and developing a therapeutic relationship is contextual (see Savage 1992, Åstedt-Kurki

& Liukkonen 1994, Mallett 1997) and part of the ongoing conversation between nurse and patient (Mallett 1997). The nurse needs an understanding of the current situation, context and patient's use of humour to ensure that any attempt at therapy is appropriate and of benefit to the patient. Much is written about the avoidance of 'negative humour' such as 'poking fun' at the patient (for example, Åstedt-Kurki & Liukkonen 1994); however, conversely, this may display and accomplish shared understandings, rapport and a customary joking relationship between participants (Norrick 1994) and nurses and patients (Mallett 1997). This is supported by findings that nurses banter with patients and humour can be produced in the form of 'mock rudeness' (Savage 1992) or teasing (Ragan 1990) and that patients may produce 'disruptive' humour to develop rapport (Mallett 1997).

Before introducing an intervention, careful assessment of the patient is necessary to ensure that humour therapy is appropriate (Simon 1989, Erdman 1991). Five criteria are useful for determining whether or not humour will be helpful. These are:

- timing – for example, humour could be considered unacceptable at the height of a crisis (although it is found during potentially difficult times – such as during gynaecological examinations [Emerson 1963, Ragan 1990]). While the value of humour is recognized by patients it should be noted that they do not always consider it to be appropriate (see Goldklang 1996, Love 1998).

- receptiveness – what might be funny to a patient at one time might not be humorous at another

- content – ensure that the patient does not find the content of the humour offensive in any way. This will be a very individual matter and is likely to vary considerably between patients

- relationship between the nurse and patient – some nurses and patients develop a 'joking relationship' which may allow for much therapeutic 'banter'; this approach will be totally inappropriate for some other patients

- patients' beliefs – some patients (and nurses) may not feel that humour and/or laughter have any place in the nurse–patient relationship and patient care.

Patients also initiate their own humour and laughter therapy to help them overcome the awfulness of their situation, such as the use of humorous videos by Cousins to reduce pain (Cousins 1976) and the use of disruptive humour to develop rapport (Mallett 1997). The nurse needs to be able to recognize the reason for the patient's use of humour and/or laughter in order to facilitate its use as a therapeutic tool.

It should be noted, however, that there is little work evaluating the use and effectiveness of humour and laughter therapy and therefore any intervention based on the suggestions above should be monitored and thoroughly evaluated similar to any other aspect of patient care.

Therapeutic potential in nursing

While there are some indications from patients and nurses that humour and/or laughter therapy is important and has potential use in patient care, further robust research is required to evaluate these interventions for appropriate use and efficacy. At present many of the potential therapeutic benefits of humour and laughter remain unproven although there is increasing evidence to support their utilization from both research results (Emerson 1963, Mallett 1997) as well as patients' accounts (Love 1998). Some possible benefits are as follows:

- to develop a therapeutic relationship between nurse and patient
- to develop rapport
- to enhance feelings of well-being
- to positively influence hopefulness
- to assist communication (including with psychiatric patients) and facilitate social interaction including –
  - to allow patients to express fears, anxieties and difficulties
  - to allow patients to raise issues
  - to avoid conflict
- to aid speech therapy
- to act as an 'icebreaker'
- to reduce pain
- to overcome the 'face-threat' of examination
- to gain and maintain patient involvement
- to facilitate patient teaching and improve recall and
- to reduce patients' anxiety.

(See also Emerson 1963, Cousins 1976, Moody 1978, Potter & Goodman 1983, Hinds et al 1984, Napora 1985, Parfitt 1990, Ragan 1990, Gaberson 1991, Hunt 1993, Mallett 1997.)

In addition, a number of studies on healthy adults indicate that humour and laughter may have specific effects which could be of benefit in, for example:

- Enhancing the immune system (Dillon et al 1985, Berk et al 1988a, 1988b)
- Increasing discomfort thresholds (Cogan et al 1987)
- Reducing muscle tension (Fry 1986)
- Assisting with cardiac and respiratory therapy (Fry 1986)
- 'Stress-buffering' (Martin & Lefcourt 1983) and coping (Coombs & Goldman 1973).

These effects may be useful within the clinical field but research is

Contraindications for use

Opinions differ on which types of humour may or may not be appropriate in therapy. This is, in part, associated with definitions of 'negative humour' (which I have taken to mean 'untherapeutic humour') – which are not always clearly elucidated or understood – and also the research methods used to gain information in this area. For example, survey research of nurses' opinions suggests that some types of what could be described as 'negative' humour – such as 'poking fun' at the patient – may not be appropriate in patient care (Åstedt-Kurki & Liukkonen 1994). However, detailed research using ethnography or conversation analysis methods of *how* humour and laughter are utilized in nurse–patient conversations indicates that some forms of banter or teasing between nurses and patients may be acceptable and appropriate (Emerson 1963, Ragan 1990, Savage 1992, Mallett 1997).

Generally the contraindications of humour are considered in terms of what humour is used to achieve. Nevertheless, the most important consideration is that humour and laughter are produced with regard to (inter alia) timing, patient receptiveness, content, nurse–patient relationship and patient's beliefs. In other words the production, appropriateness and efficacy of humour and laughter are dependent on the context in which they are produced and understood (Mallett 1997). This means that what may be therapeutic in one context is not necessarily therapeutic in another, therefore, there may be few contraindications that apply absolutely in all circumstances.

Summary

There is growing evidence from nurses, patients and other health care professionals to support humour and laughter as therapy. However, there is little research to support specific humour or laughter interventions as beneficial in the short- or long-term in the clinical environment. Humour and laughter remain potentially exciting and innovative tools for nursing therapy. They have a number of effects which could prove beneficial for many different nursing and medical diagnoses and appear to have the additional advantage of being adaptable to most situations. More clinical evaluation of humour and laughter therapy is required to fully substantiate or understand its use.

REFERENCES

Adams R M Kirkevold B 1978 Looking, smiling, laughing and moving in restaurants: sex and age differences. Environmental Psychology and Non-Verbal Behaviour 3: 117–121

Åstedt-Kurki P Liukkonen A 1994 Humor in nursing care. Journal of Advanced Nursing 20: 183–188

Åstedt-Kurki P Hopia H Vuori A 1999 Family health in everyday life: a qualitative study on well-being in families with children. Journal of Advanced Nursing 29 (3): 704–711

Berk L S Tan S A Nehlsen-Cannarella S L Napier B J Lee J W Lewis J E Hubbard R W Eby W C Fry W F 1988a Mirth modulates adrenocorticomedullary activity: suppression of cortisol and epinephrine. Clinical Research 36: 121A

Berk L S Tan S A Nehlsen-Cannarella S L Napier B J Lewis J E Lee J W Eby W C Fry W F 1988b Humor associated laughter decreases cortisol and increases spontaneous lymphocyte blastogenesis. Clinical Research 36: 435A

Berlyne D E 1972 Humor and its kin. In: Goldstein J H McGhee P E (eds) The psychology of humor. Academic Press, London, p 43–60

Bruning N 1985 Coping with chemotherapy. Dial Press, Doubleday, New York

Burkeman O 1998 You've got to laugh. The Guardian, 30 June

Chapman A J 1976 Social aspects of humorous laughter. In: Chapman A J Foot H C (eds) Humor and laughter: theory, research and applications. John Wiley, London, p 155–185

Cogan R Cogan D Waltz W McCue M 1987 Effects of laughter and relaxation on discomfort thresholds. Journal of Behavioral Medicine 10: 139–144

Coombs R H Goldman L J 1973 Maintenance and discontinuity of coping mechanisms in an intensive care unit. Social Problems 20: 342–355

Coser R L 1959 Some social functions of laughter, a study of humor in a hospital setting. Human Relations XII: 171–182

Cousins N 1976 Anatomy of an illness (as perceived by the patient). New England Journal of Medicine 295: 1458–1463

Cousins N 1979 Anatomy of an illness. Bantam, New York

Cousins N 1989 Head first the biology of hope. EP Dutton, New York

Dillon K M Minchoff B Baker K H 1985 Positive emotional states and enhancement of the immune system. International Journal of Psychiatry in Medicine 15: 13–18

Dundes A 1987 At ease, disease-AIDS jokes as sick humor. American Behavioral Scientist 30: 72–81

Dunn J R 1993 Medical perspectives on humor: an interview with William F Fry Jr. Humor & Health Journal. Jan/Feb II I (reproduced in Dunn 1999) http://www.intop.net/~jrdunn/page4.html

Emerson J P 1963 Social functions of humor in a hospital setting. PhD Thesis, University of California, Berkeley, CA

Erdman L 1991 Laughter therapy for patients with cancer. Oncology Nursing Forum 18: 1359–1363

Fosbinder D 1994 Patient perceptions of nursing care: an emerging theory of interpersonal competence. Journal of Advanced Nursing 20 (6): 1085–1093

Fry W F 1986 Humor, physiology, and the aging process. In: Nahemow L McCluskey-Fawcett K A McGhee P E (eds) Humor and aging. Academic Press, London, p 81–98

Fry W F Savin W M 1988 Mirthful laughter and blood pressure. Humor – International Journal of Humor Research 1: 49–62

Gaberson K B 1991 The effect of humorous distraction on preoperative anxiety. AORN 54: 1258–1263 (cited in Hunt 1993)

Goldklang L 1996 I'll never do a Norman Cousins. CancerOnLine Website: http://www.canceronline.org/990.20_life_goes_on.html

Goldstein J H 1982 Laugh a day, can mirth keep disease at bay? Sciences 22: 21–25

Hinds P S Martin J Vogel R J 1984 Nursing strategies to influence adolescent hopefulness during oncologic illness. Journal of Pediatric Oncology Nursing 4: 14–22 (cited in Hunt 1993)

Hunt A H 1993 Humor as a nursing intervention, Cancer Nursing 16: 34–39

Inman C E 1988 A clinic for children. MSc Dissertation, University of Warwick, Warwick, UK

Jefferson G 1984 On the organization of laughter in talk about troubles. In: Atkinson J M Heritage J (eds) Structures of social action studies in conversational analysis. Cambridge University Press, Cambridge, pp 346–369

Jefferson G Sacks H Schegloff E 1987 Notes on laughter in the pursuit of intimacy. In: Button G, Lee J R E (eds) Talk and social organisation. Multilingual Matters, Clevedon, Philadelphia, pp 152–205

Keith-Spiegel P 1972 Early conceptions of humor: varieties and issues. In: Goldstein J H McGhee P E (eds) The psychology of humor. Academic Press, London, p 3–39

Living Bible 1971 Tyndale House, UK

Love S F 1998 (revised 15/08/99) Welcome to cancer humor. CancerOnLine Website: *http://www.canceronline.org/990.20_humor_intro.html*

Mallett J 1997 Using humour. In Nurse–patient haemodialysis sessions: orchestrated institutional communication and mundane conversations. PhD Thesis, Open University, UK

Mallett J A'Hern 1996 Comparative distribution and use of humour within nurse-patient communication. International Journal of Nursing Studies 33 (5): 530–550

Martin R A Lefcourt H M 1983 Sense of humor as a moderator of the relation between stressors and moods. Journal of Personality and Social Psychology 45: 1313–1324

Moody R A 1978 Laugh after laugh, the healing power of humor. Headwaters, Florida

Napora J 1985 A study of the effects of a program of humorous activity on the subjective well-being of senior adults. Dissertation Abstracts International 46: 276–A

Nemeth P 1979 An investigation into the relationship between humor and anxiety. Dissertation Abstracts International 40: 1378–B

Norrick N R 1993 Conversational joking. Humor in everyday talk. Indiana University Press, USA

Norrick N R 1994 Involvement and joking in conversation. Journal of Pragmatics 22: 409–430

Parfitt J M 1990 Humorous preoperative teaching. AORN 52: 114–120 (cited in Hunt 1993)

Potter R E Goodman N J 1983 The implementation of laughter as a therapy facilitator with adult aphasics. Journal of Communication Disorders 16: 41–48

Ragan S L 1990 Verbal play and multiple goals in the gynaecological exam interaction. Journal of Language and Social Psychology 9 (1–2): 67–84

Robinson V 1977 Humor in nursing. In: Carlson C E Blackwell B 1977 Behavioural concepts and nursing intervention, 2nd edn. JP Lippincott, USA, p 191–210

Saltman S 1999a Kcuf Recnac Website: *http://members.aol.com/kcufrecnac/recnacmain.html*

Saltman S 1999b Kcuf Recnac Website 'Diary. Diagnosis + 6 days' *http://members.aol.com/kcufrecnac/diary/six.html*

Savage J 1992 Implications of new nursing initiatives for the nurse–patient relationship: an ethnographic study of two wards. Bloomsbury and Islington Health Authority, London

Schmitt N 1990 Patient's perception of laughter in a rehabilitation hospital. Rehabilitation Nursing 15: 143–146

Simon J 1989 Humor techniques for oncology nurses. Oncology Nursing Forum 16: 667–670

Sultanoff S M 1994 Exploring the land of mirth and funny: a voyage through the interrelationships of wit, mirth and laughter. Laugh it Up (publication of the American Association for Therapeutic Humor), p 3, reproduced in *http://www.humormatters.com.explorin.htm*

Sultanoff S M 1999 Examining the research on humor: being cautious about our conclusions. 'President's Column' in Therapeutic Humor (publication of the American Association for Therapeutic Humor, Summer) reproduced in *http://www.humormatters.com/research.html*

Treadwell D 1998 'David … I have a LUMP! Breast cancer: one husband's story'. OncoLink Website: *http://www.oncolink.upenn.edu/psychosocial/personal/survivors/story 14.html*

Warner U 1984 The serious import of humour in health visiting. Journal of Advanced Nursing 9: 83–87

Wooten P 1999a Humor cart for cancer patients. Interview with Terry Bennett. Patty Wooten's Website: *http://www.jesthealth.com/BENNETT.HTML*

Wooten P 1999b Send in the clowns! Part 1: Clown camp. Patty Wooten's Website: *http://www.jesthealth.com/SEND-C-1.HTML*

Wooten P 1999c Send in the clowns! Part 2: Caring clowning. Patty Wooten's Website: *http://www.jesthealth.com/SEND-C-2.HTML*

FURTHER READING – BOOKS

Clifford C 1996 Not Now … I'm having a no hair day: humor and healing for people with cancer. Pfeifer-Hamilton

Fox-Tennant L 1986 The effect of humor on the recovery rate of cataract patients: a pilot study. In: Nahemow L McCluskey-Fawcett K A McGhee P E (eds) Humor and aging. Academic Press, London, pp. 245–251

KEY REFERENCES

Coser R L 1959 Some social functions of laughter, a study of humour in a hospital setting. Human Relations XII: 171-182

One of the first and most important pieces of sociological humour research within a hospital environment. Uses patients' jocular talk to illustrate how humour is used, for example, to ward off danger, as a means of rebellion against authority, and as a relief from mechanical routine.

Emerson J P 1963 Social functions of humor in a hospital setting. PhD Thesis, University of California, Berkeley, CA

A seminal piece of ethnography which used participant observation to explore the use of humour between nurses and patients on an obstetrics-gynaecological ward and a medical ward in an American hospital. Emerson found that humour was spontaneous and often associated with hospital matters. Humour was used, for example, to send unofficial messages relating to death, facilitate social interaction, veil antagonism etc. Jokes were also made during the most socially invasive types of clinical examination and were related to pain, discomfort, 'loss of personal front', sexual issues etc. However, humour did not occur when patients were threatening not to cooperate or when they were very emotionally upset.

Mallett J 1997 Using humour. In Nurse–patient haemodialysis sessions: orchestrated institutional communication and mundane conversations. PhD Thesis, Open University, UK

Possibly one of the only works which uses ethnomethodological ethnography and conversation analysis approaches to study *audio-visual* video data of humour between nurses and patients learning to haemodialyse. The research indicated that humour was spontaneous, contextual, embedded in the ongoing conversation and socially organized. In addition, nurses' and patients' humour could also function simultaneously in more than one way. This included to: gain and maintain involvement; highlight anxieties and difficulties; demonstrate troubles-resistance; avoid conflict; develop rapport and disrupt thematic orientation to haemodialysis. The same data set was used to calculate the frequency and distribution of humour (Mallett & A'Hern 1996).

Ragan S L 1990 Verbal play and multiple goals in the gynaecological exam interaction. Journal of Language and Social Psychology 9 (1–2): 67–84

This is a well-executed ethnographic study of verbal play between students and a nurse practitioner in gynaecological examinations at an American university health centre. The analysis of taped audiodata indicated that shared laughter, joking and teasing occurred during the examination and the topic of humour was often associated with the process itself. Play was constructed by both participants to collude in understandings of culturally held beliefs and social mores which enable solidarity between clinician and patients and also allowed a role outside that of examiner and patient. This was thought to overcome the face threat of the examination.

Simon J M 1988 Humour and the older adult: implications for nursing. Journal of Advanced Nursing 13: 441–446

This is a correlational descriptive study of 24 adults over 61 years old from a senior citizen community centre in Texas. The research examined the relationship between the uses of humour and health outcomes as measured by perceived health, life satisfaction and morale in older adults. The findings demonstrated significant positive relationships between situational humour and perceived health and situational humour and morale, and a negative relationship between coping humour and perceived health.

USEFUL ADDRESSES AND WEBSITES

A Chuckle a Day
http://www.bright.net/~jimsjems/
usat12.htm

American Association for
Therapeutic Humor
222 S. Meramec, Suite 303
St. Louis, MO 63105, USA
Tel: +1 314 863 6232
http://aath.org

CancerOnLine
http://www.canceronline.org/

Humor and Health Institute and
Journal
PO Box 16814,
Jackson, MS 39236–6814, USA
Tel: +1 601 957 0075
E-mail: *jrdunn@intop.net*
Website: *http://www.intop.net/~jrdunn*

HumorMatters
Steven M Sultanoff
Mirthologist and Clinical
Psychologist
3972 Barranca Pkway, Suite J-221
Irvine, CA 92606, USA
Tel: +1 949 551 8839 +1 949 654 4500
E-mail:
mirthman@humormatters.com
http://www.humormatters.com/

Jest for the Health of It – Patty
Wooten *http://www.jesthealth.com/*

Kcuf Recnac
http://members.aol.com/kcufrecna
c/recnacmain.htm

International Centre for Humor and
Health
http://www.humorandhealth.com/

Nursing and Healthcare Directories
on: The Nurse Friendly Nursing
Humor
http://www.jocularity.com/

OncoLink
http://www.oncolink.upenn.edu/
psychosocial/personal/survivors

The Humor Project
110 Spring Street
Saratoga Springs
NY 12866, USA
Tel: +1 518 587 8770
http://www.humorproject.com/

25 Hypnosis

Denise Rankin-Box

Hypnosis – *the deliberate use of a trance state to enhance the sense of health and well-being.*

Trance is commonly described as an altered state of consciousness, rather like day-dreaming, when the brain appears to 'switch off' for a few seconds. This natural state may occur several times each day; however, conscious use of the trance state can help in self-healing.

Induced trance states have been used throughout the centuries and across a range of cultures and continents such as India, China and Egypt (Conachy 1994) and North America, Africa, Greece and Britain (Booth 1993). The trance state described commonly resulted from a rhythmical, repetitive activity such as swaying or dancing, as well as auditory or visual cues.

Hypnosis is the conscious use of the natural trance state and seems to provide a link with the unconscious mind through suggestion. Suggestion refers to the presentation of an idea to a client, and the extent to which the client accepts the idea (suggestibility) and is influenced by motivation and expectation. There is no definitive research to adequately explain this phemonenon. Despite this, whilst suggestion promotes a largely psychological or placebo-like response, it is possible to anaesthetize parts of the body and influence the autonomic nervous system which is not usually under voluntary control (Chakraverty et al 1992, Whorwell et al 1992).

Contrary to popular belief, the therapist does not take control of the client. In effect, all hypnosis is self-hypnosis (Vickers 1993). The therapist acts only as a facilitator and can help an individual to work towards an improvement in their health and well-being. Hypnotherapy is primarily a self-care technique and could be used, for example, in stress management, chronic and acute pain control, and management of pain during labour and dental surgery. Hypnosis can also help in resolving stammers, phobias, facial tics and habits such as smoking or overeating. However, it is important to appreciate that the client must *want* to solve their problem (Rankin Box 1995). Hypnosis may be perceived as a technique or procedure facilitating hypnotherapy as a means by which therapy is delivered.

Hypnotherapy is commonly linked with psychotherapy. Karle & Boys (1999) highlight the need for hypnotherapy to be placed into a psychotherapeutic context as a safeguard for the client who opens up repressed emotions and needs to work through them.

HISTORICAL BACKGROUND

Western recognition of hypnosis was initiated by Franz Mesmer (1734–1815) in 1773. He believed that some form of fluid could be redistributed by the force of magnetic poles. Although experiencing considerable popularity for a while, the scientific basis of this 'animal magnetism' was largely discredited and Mesmer denounced. Interest in Mesmerism was revived again in the nineteenth century, most notably by James Braid who used the term 'hypnosis'. Braid suggested that Mesmer's clients had been in a trance state which could be induced in a number of ways such as watching a swinging pendulum or staring at a distant point or light (Booth 1993). Braid called this 'neurohypnotism' from the Greek *hypnos* meaning sleep since he thought that the trance state induced a neurological response similar to but different from sleep.

During World War I, Simmel developed a technique called 'hypno-analysis' for treating war neurosis (Tamin 1988). More recent developments in this field are described by Erickson & Rossi (1980) and Spiegel & Spiegel (1978). Hypnotism is gaining popularity in health care and has been recommended for study by the British and American Medical Associations (Booth 1993). According to Woodham & Peters (1997), despite being tainted by the exploits of showmen, hypnotherapy is actually supported by more scientific research than many other complementary therapies.

TREATMENT

Initially the therapist takes a general history from the client and identifies problems of current concern. Trance induction can take many forms and therapists may choose a technique to suit the client. Commonly, subjects are asked to focus on a point and let their breathing become slow and regular. As their eyelids become heavy, they are asked to close them and start to relax. The clients control the extent to which they relax into the trance state.

Guided visualization techniques such as imagining a walk along a beach or in a garden are practised with caution since they may not always trigger a positive response; for example, strong images of summer days have been known to initiate asthma attacks and an imaginary tour around a house could induce claustrophobia. It may be preferable to ask the client to imagine a scene or a place in which they would feel contented and relaxed.

A therapist ends the trance state gradually, allowing the client to control the speed at which he emerges from the trance state. Reorientation may be facilitated by the therapist counting back from three to one.

Descriptions of the trance state vary from an altered state of consciousness similar to a meditative state to a heightened sense of awareness. It is not uncommon for individuals to feel very relaxed or have sensations of heaviness or lightness. The hypnotherapist's voice may fade away as the client becomes more relaxed. As with any therapy, it is important to ensure you choose a qualified professional practitioner.

Stages of technique

Induction – commonly linked to a relaxation technique.

Trigger – may be used to enable deeper relaxed states to occur by suggestion.

Deepening (ideo-motor response) – refers to client's response to questions using, for example, finger movement rather than a spoken reply, to facilitate deeper relaxation.

Therapy – the stage where the client's concerns are addressed, e.g. becoming less anxious, more assertive, ego-boosting.

Lightener/reorientation – the client is gently reorientated with his surroundings before coming out of the trance state.

Ending – the client is reorientated and commonly it is suggested that he will come out of trance after counting from 3 to 1.

Therapeutic potential in nursing

Some examples of potential applications of hypnosis in nursing practice are as follows:

- Relaxation
- Acute and chronic pain management
- Childbirth – management of labour pain
- Stress management
- Control of certain phobias – needle phobia during, for example, renal dialysis, chemotherapy, diabetes
- Post-amputation phantom pain management
- Relief of nausea during pregnancy, drug treatment or postoperatively
- In casualty simple trance techniques may be used to relax or 'numb' an area requiring suturing – this can be effective in both children and adults

Therapeutic potential in nursing (Cont'd)

- Insomnia
- Hypertension
- Irritable bowel syndrome
- Self-hypnosis – taught to clients for pain control in labour, acute anxiety attacks, insomnia, relaxation and so on.

Contraindications for use

- Whilst hypnosis can be extremely valuable it is important that the therapist is competent to deal with the particular problem.
- Avoid long-standing psychological problems which may require professional counselling/treatment.
- Occasionally clients may feel lightheaded when coming out of a deep trance state and it important to know how to manage this and any abreactions that may occur.
- Avoid hypnotherapy or self-hypnosis if the patient has severe depression, epilepsy or psychosis.

Summary

Hypnosis has considerable potential for use within nursing practice. The possible applications are wide-ranging and it is a therapy which gives clients responsibility for their own healing. Whether it can be used effectively in the clinical setting depends largely on clients' willingness to manage their own health care; the therapist acts only as a facilitator of the healing process.

REFERENCES

Booth B 1993 Complementary therapy. Nursing Times/Macmillan, London
Chakraverty K et al 1992 Erythromyalgia: the role of hypnotherapy. Postgraduate Medical Journal 68: 44–46
Conachy S 1994 Hypnotherapy. In: Wells R Tschudin V (eds) Wells' supportive therapies in health care. Baillière Tindall, London
Erickson M Rossi E 1980 (eds) Innovative hypnotherapy – the collected papers of Milton H. Erickson on hypnosis. Irvington, New York, vol IV
Karle H Boys J 1999 Hypnotherapy: a practical handbook. Free Association Books, London
Rankin-Box D F 1995 Hypnosis. In: Rankin-Box D F (ed) The nurses' handbook of complementary therapies, 1st edn. Churchill Livingstone, Edinburgh, pp 119–124

Spiegel H Spiegel D 1978 Trance and treatment: clinical uses of hypnosis. Basic Books, New York

Tamin J 1988 Hypnosis. In: Rankin-Box D F (ed) Complementary health therapies: a guide for nurses and the caring professions. Croom Helm, Beckenham, Kent, pp 189–202

Vickers A 1993 Complementary medicine and disability: alternatives for people with disabling conditions. Chapman and Hall, London

Whorwell P J et al 1992 Physiological effects of emotion: assessment via hypnosis. Lancet 340: 69–72

Woodham A Peters D 1997 The encyclopedia of complementary medicine. Dorling Kindersley, London

FURTHER READING – JOURNALS

Chakraverty K et al 1992 Erythromyalgia: the role of hypnotherapy. Postgraduate Medical Journal 68: 44–46

Chapman L F Goodell H Wolff H G 1959 Changes in tissue vulnerability induced during hypnotic suggestion. Journal of Psychosomatic Research 4: 99–105

Contach P Hockenbury M Herman S 1985 Self-hypnosis as antiemetic therapy in children receiving chemotherapy. Oncology Nursing Forum 12: 41–46

Ewer T C Stewart D E 1986 Improvement of bronchial hyperresponsiveness in patients with moderate asthma after treatment with a hypnotic technique: a randomised controlled trial. British Journal of Medicine (Clinical Research) 293: 1129–1132

Holroyd J Hill A 1989 Pushing the limits of recovery: hypnotherapy with a stroke patient. International Journal of Clinical and Experimental Hypnosis 37: 120–128

Maslach C Marshall G Zimbardo P G 1972 Hypnotic control of peripheral skin temperature: a case report. Psychophysiology 9. 600–605

Minichello W E 1987 Treatment of hyperhidrosis of amputation site with hypnosis and suggestions involving classical conditioning. International Journal of Psychosomatics 34: 7–8

Negley-Parker E Araoz D L 1986 Hypnotherapy with families of chronically ill children. International Journal of Psychosomatics 33: 9–11

Whorwell P J et al 1992 Physiological effects of emotion: assessment via hypnosis. Lancet 340: 69–72

FURTHER READING – BOOKS

Bandler R 1985 Using your brain for a change. Real People Press, Utah

Garner G Olness K (eds) 1981 Hypnosis and hypnotherapy with children. Grune & Stratton, New York

Hartland J 1971 Medical and dental hypnosis. Baillière Tindall, London

Rosen S (ed) 1982 My voice will go with you: the teaching tales of Milton Erickson. WW Norton, London

Spiegel H Spiegel D 1978 Trance and treatment: clinical uses of hypnosis. Basic Books, New York

Young P 1987 Personal change through self-hypnosis. Angus and Robertson, London

USEFUL ADDRESSES

At present there are no nationally accredited courses in hypnosis. The Institute of Complementary Medicine maintains a register of hypnotherapists affiliated to professional organizations.

British Association of Therapeutical Hypnotists (BATH)
Belmont Centre
46 Belmont Road
Ramsgate
Kent CT11 7QG
Tel: 0184 358 7927

British Hypnotherapy Association
67, Upper Berkeley Street,
London W1H 5W1
Tel: 0171 723 4443

British Society of Experimental and Clinical Hypnosis
c/o Phyllis Alden
Department of Psychology
Grimsby General Hospital
Scartho Road
Grimsby
South Humberside DN33 2BA

British Society of Medical and Dental Hypnosis
National Office
17 Keppel View Road
Kimberworth
Rotherham
South Yorkshire S61 2AR

British Society of Medical and Dental Hypnosis (Scotland)
PO Box 1007
Glasgow G31 2LE

Central Register of Advanced Hypnotherapists
PO Box 14526
London N4 2WG

Institute of Complementary Medicine
PO Box 194
London SE16 1QZ

The National College for Hypnosis and Psychotherapy
12 Cross Street, Nelson
Lancs BB9 7EN

Therapy Training College
10 Balaclava Road
Kings Health
Birmingham B14 7SG
Tel: 0121 444 5435

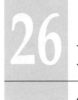

26 Massage

Carol Horrigan

Massage – *a conscious, deliberate, and often formalized use of the instinctive response to comfort another person using touch.*

The many systems of massage practised now in the UK have all been adopted from other cultures. They can be stimulating or sedating, vigorous or gentle and include all or part of the patient's body; they may be performed using the practitioner's hands, feet, elbows or knees as well as instruments or machines. Some methods use oil, cream or a lotion to lubricate the skin; for others, talcum powder is preferred. If possible, the patient lies on a couch or bed, although some therapists prefer to work on a thin mattress or rug on the floor. Massage does not have to include the whole body or take more than an hour to complete. Apart from this being impractical for a nurse massage therapist, many patients are too unwell to tolerate more than 10–20 minutes of massage and this is usually sufficient to achieve the desired effect. Massage can usually be adapted to the circumstances and comfort of the patient. For example, if a patient is breathless when lying down or if they spend most of their day in a wheelchair.

British people have a reputation for being reserved and touch or caress is considered a private and intimate activity, often linked with sex. Foreign travel and immigrants from other cultures have helped to create a more relaxed society in which physical expressions of gratitude or affection are becoming acceptable. Massage as a therapeutic intervention is rapidly gaining recognition.

Many claims are made for the effects of massage. Some of these have been investigated and upheld by research (Acolet et al 1993, Adamson, 1996, Porter 1996, Graydon & McKee 1997, Byass 1999) regarding physiological changes; other claims are in contention (Barr & Taslitz 1970, Reed & Held 1988, Ferrel-Torry & Glick 1993); but many have remained empirically anecdotal for thousands of years, and need substantiation for the now evidence-based profession of nursing. Quantitative research commonly measures physiological changes but massage creates quality of life effects which are difficult to measure. However, research is in progress, especially that being carried out as part of MA and MSc degrees in bodywork offered by UK universities.

HISTORICAL BACKGROUND

The word massage derives from Arabic, Greek, Hindi and French words associated with touch, pressing or shampooing. Both the Bible and the Koran refer to anointing the skin with oil (Beck 1988). Documents (in the British Museum) describe massage being performed around 3000 BC in China. Various techniques were refined by the Japanese and Middle Eastern cultures as part of their health and hygiene routines. The Greeks and Romans used massage to prepare soldiers and gladiators. However, in the Middle Ages religious dogma and supersition regarded anything related to physical or emotional pleasure as sinful. Not until the Renaissance did a renewed interest in aesthetics and health reinstate massage as a beneficial activity.

In 1870, massage was introduced to the United States from Europe, and in 1884 the first book on the subject was published there. That same year, a group of women in England formed the Society of Trained Masseuses which later became the Chartered Society of Physiotherapists (1964). During both World Wars massage was used in the rehabilitation of injured men. Archives at the University College and Middlesex Schools of Nursing show that nurses were being trained in massage in the early twentieth century. However, the increased use of technology led to a decline in the use of massage by both nurses and physiotherapists. There has been a gradual resurgence of massage in nursing since the 1970s. Beginning in the care of the elderly and care of the dying, it is gaining recognition now in all nursing specialties.

TREATMENT

Massage, like any other intervention, needs to be planned following an assessment of the patient and evaluated when it has been implemented. Preparations for massage should include the following:

- Identifying the problems that massage may be able to relieve
- Ascertaining positions that the patient may or may not be able to adopt
- Checking that all medications/interventions are completed for the period of the massage
- Making sure the patient is comfortable (bladder, bowels, respiratory function, pain control)
- Ensuring the massage will be undisturbed (single room, 'do not disturb' sign)

- Having adequate facilities (heating, towels, pillows, adjustable bed, comfortable chair)
- Explaining the rationale for massage to the patient/relatives and proceeding only if they agree to it (Baldwin 1986, De Wever 1977).

The rhythmic movement of massage is comforting and relaxing, and the patient will want to rest afterwards. Lifting equipment or colleagues to help with any transfer should be arranged before the massage to avoid disrupting its relaxing effects.

The therapist will adjust every massage session to suit the patient's needs, desires and tolerance, but some measures and processes are almost always included:

- The therapist prepares (in her preferred way) to ensure a calm frame of mind; all other responsibilities are accounted for, and an assessment of the patient is made.
- The working area is prepared with adequate heating, 'do not disturb' signs, towels, blankets, pillows and massage oil.
- The patient is made comfortable and covered with towels to expose only the part of the body being massaged, so that dignity and warmth are maintained at all times.
- Massage begins and ends with slow, stroking movements (effleurage); this ensures a sense of calm and relaxation.
- A range of massage movements and gentle passive exercise of the muscles or joints is carried out in a logical order, according to the style of massage being used.
- Finally, the patient is warmly covered, the therapist indicates that treatment is completed and the patient is left to rest.

Therapeutic potential in nursing

Research has indicated that massage can have the following beneficial effects:

- Reduction in anxiety levels (Acolet 1993, Field et al 1993, Fraser & Ross Kerr 1993)
- Emotional stress relief (Longworth 1982, McKecknie 1983)
- Relief of muscular tension and fatigue (Balke et al 1989)
- Improved local and distant lymphatic circulation (Morgan et al 1992, Mortimer 1990)
- Better local blood circulation, leading to a feeling of warmth (Hovind & Neilsen 1974, Kaada & Torsteinbo 1989)
- Pain relief due to the release of endorphins, leading to relaxation (Kaada & Torsteinbo 1989).

Contraindications for use

- Extremes of body temperature
  - if a patient is hypothermic, massage may increase surface circulation and seriously reduce core temperature
  - the same mechanism would exacerbate the discomfort of the patient with pyrexia who also may not wish to be touched
- Contagious diseases/acute infections
  - besides disturbing body temperature, there is the danger of disease transmission
- Acute, undiagnosed back pain
  - this may be simple muscular spasm or potentially dangerous compression of the spinal cord; no massage should be carried out until a diagnosis has been made
- Fractures
  - massage cannot be carried out directly over fracture sites but it is useful, when applied to other areas of the body, for relaxing orthopaedic patients
- Cardiovascular instability (hypertension, angina, cardiac oedema)
  - massage is beneficial only if given in short, non-tiring sessions
- Respiratory insufficiency
  - patients may need to remain sitting upright during massage and this can be arranged
- Deep vein thrombosis – *never massage feet, legs or trunk*
  - very light hand or face massage will not increase circulation enough to move emboli, and may reduce patient's anxiety
- Varicose veins/phlebitis
  - massage here requires a specialized technique, not taught by most massage schools. Standard pressures and movements may induce itching, causing the patient to scratch and accidentally damage the veins
- Low platelet count and other causes of easy bruising
  - this includes patients with leukaemia, purpura, and those receiving chemotherapy, radiotherapy, or high-dose anticoagulant therapy
  - provided the massage is very gentle and care is taken when massaging over bony prominences, the patient will benefit
- Unexplained lumps and bumps
  - these should be diagnosed before massage
- Unstable pregnancy
  - Massage should not be given to the abdomen, legs and feet for the first trimester
- Cancer patients
  - metastases are not caused or spread by gentle surface massage (McNamara 1993)
  - chemotherapy and radiotherapy may make the skin very dry
  - some radiologists will not permit massage to areas currently undergoing radiotherapy

Contraindications for use (Cont'd)

- — lymphoedema requires a special type of massage and should not be attempted by the untrained
- ■ Chronic fatigue syndrome
  - — patients can usually only tolerate short treatments when the syndrome is active
- ■ People with HIV/AIDS
  - — many of the conditions above will apply
  - — loss of weight and/or Karposi's sarcoma may make massage uncomfortable unless a gentle touch and extra lubricant are used
- ■ Dermatology patients
  - — very few skin diseases are contagious, but infection is a risk if the patient has broken skin
- ■ Rheumatoid arthritis and osteoarthrosis
  - — careful positioning of the patient and frequent change of position may be required
- ■ Dementia and psychosis
  - — such patients may be confused or frightened by massage and its effects
- ■ Contact lenses
  - — some types should not be worn with the eyes shut; check that the patient has removed them.

Summary

Massage can be used in nursing from its simplest form of hand massage with lotion to advanced techniques for symptom control. For the patient it is a welcome contrast to the technological procedures of modern medicine.

Touch is an integral aspect of communication and nursing care where the use of massage can promote a relaxing and therapeutic environment.

REFERENCES

Acolet D et al 1993 Changes in plasma cortisol and catecholamine concentrations in response to massage in pre-term infants. Archives of Disease in Childhood 68: 29–31

Adamson S 1996 Teaching baby massage to new parents. Complementary Therapies in Nursing and Midwifery 2: 151–159

Baldwin L C 1986 The therapeutic use of touch with the elderly. Physical and Occupational Therapy in Geriatrics 4: 45–50

Balke B Anthony J Wyatt F 1989 The effects of massage treatment on exercise fatigue. Clinical Sports Medicine 1: 189–196

Barr J S Taslitz N 1970 The influence of back massage on autonomic functions. Physical Therapy 50: 1679–1691

Beck M 1988 The theory and practice of therapeutic massage. Milady, New York

Byass R 1999 Auditing complementary therapies in palliative care. Complementary Therapies in Nursing & Midwifery 5: 51–60

De Weaver M K 1977 Nursing home patients' perceptions of nurses' affective touching. Journal of Psychology 96: 163–171

Ferrel-Torry A T Glick O J 1993 The use of therapeutic massage as a nursing intervention to modify anxiety and the perception of cancer pain. Cancer Nursing 16: 93–101

Field T M et al 1993 Tactile/kinaesthetic stimulation. Paediatrics 77: 654–658

Fraser J Ross Kerr J 1993 Psychophysiological effects of back massage in elderly institutionalised patients. Journal of Advanced Nursing 18: 238–245

Grayon J McKee N 1997 Massage therapy for patients with multiple sclerosis. International Journal of Alternative & Complementary Medicine July: 27–28

Hovind H Neilsen S L 1974 Effect of massage on blood flow in skeletal muscle. Scandinavian Journal of Rehabilitation Medicine 6: 74–77

Kaada B Torsteinbo O 1989 Increase of plasma beta endorphin levels in connective tissue massage. General Pharmacology 20: 487–489

Longworth J C D 1982 Psychophysiological effects of slow stroke massage in normotensive females. Advances in Nursing Science July: 44–46

McKecknie A A et al 1983 Anxiety states: a preliminary report on the value of connective tissue massage. Journal of Psychosomatic Research 27: 125–129

McNamara P 1993 Massage for people with cancer. Wandsworth Cancer Support Centre, London

Morgan R G et al 1992 Complex physical therapy for the lymphoedematous arm. Journal of Hand Surgery 178: 437–441

Mortimer P S 1990 The measurement of skin lymph flow by isotope clearance – reliability, reproducibility, injection dynamics and the effect of massage. Journal of Investigative Dermatology 95: 677–681

Porter S J 1996 The use of massage for neonates requiring special care. Complementary Therapies in Nursing & Midwifery 2: 93–95

Reed B V Held J M 1988 Effects of sequential connective tissue massage on the autonomic nervous system of middle aged and elderly adults. Physical Therapy 68: 1231–1234

FURTHER READING – JOURNALS

Barnet K 1972 A theoretical construct of the concepts of touch as they relate to nursing. Nursing Research 21: 102–110

Corner J Crawley N Hildebrand S 1995 An evaluation of the use of massage and essential oils on the wellbeing of cancer patients. International Journal of Palliative Nursing 1 (12): 67–73

Jackson S 1985 The touching process in rehabilitation. Australian Nurses' Journal 14: 43–45

Nalkin K 1994 Use of massage in clinical practice. British Journal of Nursing 3 (6): 292–294

Wilkinson S 1995 Aromatherapy and massage in palliative care. International Journal of Palliative Nursing 1 (1): 21–30

FURTHER READING – BOOKS

Dawes N Harrold F 1990 Massage cures. Thorsons, Wellingborough

Maxwell-Hudson C 1988 The complete book of massage. Dorling Kindersley, London

Montague A 1986 Touching – the human significance of the skin, 3rd edn. Harper & Row, New York

USEFUL ADDRESSES

Clare Maxwell-Hudson's Massage
Training Centre
PO Box 457
London NW2 4BR
Tel: 0181 450 6494

Northern Institute of Massage
100 Waterloo Road
Blackpool
Lancashire FY4 1AW
Tel: 01253 403548

The Raworth Centre
20–26 South Street

Dorking
Surrey RH 42HQ
Tel: 01306 742150

For first and high degrees in
bodywork or massage:
University of Westminster
The Admissions and Marketing
Office
Cavendish Campus
115 New Cavendish Street
London W1M 8JS
Tel: 020 7911 5000

Other Universities also have diploma and degree courses available. Enquiries should be made directly to the individual campus.

27 Music as therapy

Francis C Biley

Music as therapy – *the use of music in the accomplishment of therapeutic aims: the restoration, maintenance and improvement of mental and physical health* (Bunt 1994)

The definition above is not to be confused with a slightly different definition of *music therapy* which involves 'a systematic process of intervention wherein the therapist helps the client to achieve health using musical experiences and the relationships that develop through them as dynamic forces of change' (Bruscia, 1989). It could be argued that there is little difference between these two definitions. However, while *music therapy* can only be performed by a qualified music therapist, *music as therapy* can be used informally or more formally by nurses, midwives, other health care professionals, patients and clients to achieve quite significant improvements in happiness, health and well-being.

The use of music as therapy can take a very wide variety of forms. Informally, music can be used for background listening, where back ground music is played, and listened to, in a wide variety of acute health care environments, clinics, long-term care facilities or our own homes. Many of us are using music in this way when we turn on the car radio while driving or the hi-fi after a busy day at work. More formally, music can be employed in a therapeutic capacity in music listening group sessions, live concerts, or participation in the creation of music, such as musical groups employing traditional (Western) instruments or by chanting, praying, reciting a mantra or drumming. In this chapter the therapeutic potential of listening to music with the aim of promoting relaxation and stress reduction will be explored.

HISTORICAL BACKGROUND

There is evidence that musical instruments existed many thousands of years ago (McClellan 1991) when our earliest ancestors attributed magical powers to sound (McClellan 1991, Cowan 1992). They 'used music in the form of incantations, songs, rhythms, and sounds to ward off evil spirits, absolve sins, or placate the Gods' (Alvin 1966). In ancient Egypt, music was regarded as the 'physic of the soul' (Cook

1981) and elsewhere in early history healers were often also musicians (Heitz et al 1992). Beck (1991) stated that Plato believed that music had the ability to promote health in body and mind. Homer thought that music could help to avoid negative feelings such as sadness, anger, worry and fear (Cook 1981).

Many centuries later music was used to treat the mental health problems of notable figures such as King Philip V of Spain, King Ludwig II of Bavaria and King George II of Great Britain (Podalsky 1954).

Early experiments into the therapeutic use of music were published by Pargiter in the eighteenth century (Buckwalter et al 1985) and Dogiel in 1830 (cited in Campbell 1991). The latter suggested that physiological responses to music included an influence on the circulation of blood. The first book on the subject was written by Dr Hector Chomat in 1846 (Alvin 1966, cited by Cook 1981). This may have prompted Florence Nightingale to recognize the potential importance of music in caring for the sick. In 1859 she wrote that 'wind instruments, including the human voice, and stringed instruments ... have generally a beneficial effect ... an air ... will sensibly soothe [the sick]' (Nightingale 1859).

Results showing that the blood circulation to the brain was slowed and reduced by the effects of music were published by Patrici in 1896 (Walters 1954, cited by Cook 1981). Further research performed early in the twentieth century showed that by 1926 there was 'agreement that music effectively increases metabolism; changes muscular energy; accelerates respiration; produces marked but variable effects on volume, pulse and blood pressure; creates the physiological basis for the genesis of emotional shifts' (Campbell 1991).

Perhaps as a result of some of these findings, the first schools of Music Therapy were opened during the 1940s in Michigan State University and the University of Kansas (Cook 1981). More recently there has been a revival in the use of music as therapy and a considerable amount of research is being performed in order to establish potential benefits.

TREATMENT

Treatment, in music listening terms, consists simply of listening to music. However, a number of issues need to be taken into account. In the strictest sense, if any recorded music is to be played publicly, then licences from the Performing Rights Society and Phonographic Performance Limited need to be obtained. Equipment that will allow good quality music reproduction, or in other words that will sound good, needs to be obtained and the music needs to be chosen. According to Stevens (1990), 'the therapeutic benefits of music relate strongly to the type and character of the music being played'. With this in mind, in order to promote relaxation and stress reduction, it is important to choose music that uses no predominant percussion (Kaempf & Amodei 1989), that is primarily created by stringed instruments (White 1992), is low-pitched (White 1992) and predictable with a tempo of about 60–80 beats per minute. Harvey (1987) found that New Age and classical music was more consistent than other forms of music in inducing positive alterations in physiological states. Taking individual choice and preferences into account, classical music such as Pachelbel's 'Canon in D', Vaughan Williams' 'Lark Ascending' and Handel's 'Water Music' may be considered ideal music for relaxation. Similarly, a wide variety of New Age music that has been written specifically for the purposes of relaxation is available, much of which is suitable.

Contraindications for use

- When listening to music for therapeutic purposes, the choice of music is critical. What might be relaxing or diversionary for one individual might not be for the next.

- Music preferences can be strongly age- and cultural background-specific and these issues need to be taken into account when choosing music

- Hearing a specific piece of music may trigger unpleasant prior associations for an individual

- There is evidence to suggest that listening to music with negative, aggressive or violent lyrics, as typified by the heavy metal genre, may have perceived negative effects on individuals (McCraty et al 1998). However, on the whole, it is unlikely that participation in music listening or any other more active music participation has any great potential risk when compared to, for example, having a surgical procedure, receiving anaesthesia, or any of a range of alternative and complementary therapies.

Therapeutic potential in nursing

- Research indicates consistent improvements in the psychological state of study participants upon exposure to music (Barnason et al 1995)

- Music may promote stress reduction and relaxation (Hanser 1988)

- There are indicators that there are positive responses to music obtained from variables such as pulse rate, blood pressure, electroencephalograph and galvanic skin response (Thaut 1990, Watkins 1997)

- Individualized selection of music to listen to post-medical intervention may act as a displacement tool reducing feelings of fear and uncertainty (Stevens 1990)

Therapeutic potential in nursing (cont'd)

- Music therapy and relaxation therapy can be effective in reducing stress in post-myocardial infarction patients (Guzzetta 1989)
- Music therapy encourages individuals to shift their perceptions of time into two types – virtual and experimental. Virtual time, perceived in left brain mode, is characterized by hours, minutes and seconds. Experiential time is perceived through the memory and right brain mode (Brewer 1998)
- Slow-moving music lengthens our perception of time because the memory has more time to experience the events and the spaces between the events (Brewer 1998). This results in a distortion of the individual's perception of time, encouraging and enabling individuals to reduce anxiety, fear and pain (McClellan 1979)
- Music therapy can help patients achieve a state of relaxation, increased self-awareness and creativity (Hamel 1979)
- Music can reduce feelings of fear and anxiety
- The use of calming music during labour and childbirth as a displacement tactic is well established although there is little research to substantiate its use.

Summary

Music as therapy can be defined as 'the use of music in the accomplishment of therapeutic aims: the restoration, maintenance and improvement of mental and physical health' (Bunt 1994) and it can take a very wide variety of forms. For thousands of years and in many different settings, music has been used as a part of a healing process. While the research on the value of music as a therapeutic intervention is inconclusive, it does seem as though 'individuals in stressful situations, such as the hospital or dental environment, respond to music in a positive way ...' (Hanser 1988).

REFERENCES

Aldridge D 1994 An overview of music therapy research. Complementary Therapies in Medicine 2(4): 204–216

Alvin J 1996 Music therapy. J Baker, London

Bampton P Draper P 1997 The effects of relaxation music on patient tolerance of gastrointestinal endoscopic procedures. Journal of Clinical Gastroenterology 25(1): 343–345

Barnason S Zimmerman L Nieveen J 1995 The effects of music intervention on anxiety in the patient after coronary artery bypass grafting. Heart and Lung 24(2): 124–132

Beck S L 1991 The therapeutic use of music for cancer-related pain. Oncology Nursing Forum 18 (8): 1327–1337

Brewer J F 1998 Healing sounds. Complementary Therapies in Nursing & Midwifery 4(1): 7–12

Bruscia K E 1989 Defining music therapy. Springhouse, Pennsylvania

Buckwalter K Hartsock J Gaffney J 1985 Music therapy. In: Bulecheck G M McCloskey J C (eds) Nursing interventions: treatments for nursing diagnosis. W B Saunders, Philadelphia

Bunt L 1994 Music therapy: an art beyond words. Routledge, London

Cowan J G 1992 The Aborigine tradition. Element, Dorset

Good M 1996 Effects of relaxation and music on postoperative pain: a review. Journal of Advanced Nursing 24(5): 905–914

Guzzetta C E 1989 The effects of relaxation and music therapy on patients in a coronary care unit with presumptive acute M.I. Heart and Lung 18 (6): 609

Hamel M P 1979 Through music to self. Shambhala Press, Boulder, CO

Hanser S B 1988 Controversy in music listening/Stress Reduction Research. The Arts in Psychotherapy 15: 211–217

Harvey A 1987 Music and health. USA Today, 17 December: 9–11

Heitz L Symreng T Scamman F L 1992 Effect of music therapy in the Post-anaesthesia care unit: a nursing intervention. Journal of Post Anaesthesia Nursing 7(1): 22–31

Iwanaga M Tsukamoto M 1997 Effects of excitative and sedative music on subjective and physiologic relaxation. Perceptual and Motor Skills 85(1): 287–296

Kaempf G Amodei M E 1989 The effects of music on anxiety. Association of Operating Room Nurses Journal 50 (1): 112–118

McClellan R 1991 The healing forces of music: history, theory and practice. Element, Massachusetts

McCraty R Barrios-Chopin B Atkinson M Tomasino D 1998 The effects of different types of music on mood, tension, and mental clarity. Alternative Therapies in Health and Medicine 4(1): 75–84

Nightingale F 1859 Notes on nursing: what it is and what it is not. Reprinted in 1969 by Dover Publications, New York

Podalsky E 1954 Music therapy. Philosophical Library, New York

Ragneskog H Kihlgren M 1997 Music and other strategies to improve the care of agitated patients with dementia. Interviews with experienced staff. Scandinavian Journal of Caring Sciences 11(3): 176–182

Stevens K M 1990 Patients' perceptions of music during surgery. Journal of Advanced Nursing 15: 1045–1051

Thaut M H 1990 Physiological and motor responses to music stimuli. In: Unkefer R F (ed) Music Therapy in the Treatment of Adults with Mental Disorders. Schirmer Books, New York

Walters 1954 How music produces its effects on the brain and mind. In: Podalsky E (ed) Music Therapy. Philosophical Library, New York

Watkins G R 1997 Music therapy: proposed physiological mechanisms and clinical implications. Clinical Nurse Specialist 11 (2): 43–50

White J M 1992 Music therapy: an intervention to reduce anxiety in the myocardial patient. Clinical Nurse Specialist 6(2): 58–63

FURTHER READING – JOURNALS

Aldridge D 1994 An overview of music therapy research. Complementary Therapies in Medicine 2(4): 204–216
Hanser S B 1988 Controversy in music listening/stress reduction research. The Arts in Psychotherapy 15: 211–217

FURTHER READING – BOOKS

Aldridge D 1996 Music therapy research and practice in medicine: from out of the silence. Jessica Kingsley, London
Newman P 1997 Therapeutic voicework: principles and practice for the use of singing as a therapy. Jessica Kingsley, London

USEFUL ADDRESSES

British Society for Music Therapy
Roehampton Institute London
Digby Stuart College
Roehampton Lane
London SW15 5PU
http://www.roehampton.ac.uk/
artshum/bsmt/bsmt.htm

American Music Therapy
Association

8455 Colesville Road, Suite 1000
Silver Spring, Maryland 20910, USA
http://www.musictherapy.org

The Tomatis Method
Tomatis International
6 Place de la République
Dominicaine
75017 Paris, France
http://www.tomatis.com

28 Naturopathy

Brian Isbell

Naturopathy – *a multidisciplinary approach to health care founded on the belief in the power of the body to heal itself.*

There are many systems of naturopathy practised in the UK but they all share a common philosophy. The aims are to maintain health by supporting and stimulating the *vis medicatrix naturae* (the healing power of nature). Naturopaths share the belief that only nature can cure. Four basic principles of naturopathy are:

- the individual is unique
- establish the cause(s) of the condition rather than treat the symptom(s)
- individuals possess the power to heal themselves
- treat the whole person and not only the area of body affected.

Naturopathic approaches stress the importance of health maintenance, disease prevention as well as patient education. Naturopaths believe that the body will always strive towards good health, the establishment of homeostasis and is its own best healer (Woodham & Peters 1997). Naturopathy is an approach to health rather than a specific therapy and emphasizes a way of life that is in harmony with nature (Featherstone & Forsyth 1997).

Most naturopaths in the UK base their treatment on the assessment of the correct diet and nutrients for the individual, adequate rest and relaxation, exercise, fresh air, clean water and sunlight. Many naturopaths therefore utilize treatments which include dietary advice, in some cases including the use of supplements, detoxification methods, bodywork (e.g. massage or osteopathy), hydrotherapy, counselling and advice on lifestyle. Naturopaths may use herbal medicine or homeopathy and in addition some use acupuncture. Particularly naturopaths trained in the USA, Australia or New Zealand are eclectic in their approach and use a wide range of natural therapies with the aim to stimulate the body's ability to heal itself. No matter how diverse the range of treatments used by the naturopath the treatment methods and plan are tailored to the unique needs of the patient.

HISTORICAL BACKGROUND

Some aspects of naturopathy share a common ground with some of the ancient holistic health systems such as Ayurveda and Traditional Chinese Medicine (Woodham & Peters 1997). In these holistic systems all aspects of the patient are considered and treatment approaches take into account the physical type, diet, exercise, rest and the relaxation requirements of the individual. Such approaches mirror the holistic philosophy of naturopathy in which the physical, biochemical, environmental, hereditary and psychological aspects of the individual are taken into account.

Many of the principles of naturopathy are based on the teachings of the Greek physician, Hippocrates (c 460–375 BC) who is considered as the 'father of medicine'. Hippocrates established the principle that practitioners should 'first do no harm'. In his teachings he maintained that health was dependent upon eating simple good quality food and on exercising, and that disease occurred as a result of a disturbance of the balance of the body. The loss of balance Hippocrates stated should be treated in accordance with natural laws. Essentially in his teachings he claimed only nature heals and it must be given the opportunity to do so. He taught that frequently what is considered to be disease in fact is an expression of purification where the body is attempting to eliminate unwanted or toxic materials by fevers, sweating or swellings (inflammation), vomiting or diarrhoea. His teachings emphasized that these symptoms must not be suppressed as they are the methods by which the patient's body is attempting to eliminate toxins.

The term naturopathy was first used in the nineteenth century. During this period systems of nature cures were developed both in the USA and Europe. The approaches included the natural methods of hydrotherapy, fasting, fresh air, good quality drinking water, sunlight and exercise.

Naturopathy is now practised on many continents. In some US states naturopaths are recognized as primary care physicians (Micozzi 1996). In Germany, Heilpraktiker (health practitioners) are state licensed. In other countries such as the UK, Canada, South Africa, Israel, Australia and New Zealand naturopaths enjoy a degree of autonomy (Woodham & Peters 1997).

TREATMENT

Naturopaths, especially eclectic practitioners, use a wide range of natural therapies. For further details on the nature of treatments used reference should be made to other chapters of this book (Acupuncture chapter 15;, Communication Skills and Counselling, chpater 20; Herbal

Medicine, chapter 22; Homeopathy, chpater 23; Massage, chapter 26; Osteopathy, chpater 29; and Relaxation and Visualization, chapter 31).

Consideration of the therapeutic potential of such a diverse group of therapies indicates the extensive range of conditions for which naturopathy may be beneficial. At one end of the spectrum there are practitioners who adhere closely to the 'nature cure' tradition that is focused on diet, detoxification, hydrotherapy, counselling and lifestyle advice. At the other end of the spectrum there are eclectic practitioners who in addition use a wide range of therapies including pharmaceutical-grade botanical medicines (Micozzi 1996). Naturopaths therefore have much to offer particularly in the treatment of degenerative and chronic conditions such as arthritis and asthma, while consideration of the mind–body dimension has led to naturopathy being used in the treatment of patients with chronic fatigue (Peters et al 1996) or depression. The emphasis on analysis of the diet and nutrient needs of the individual means that patients with gastrointestinal problems, including 'leaky' gut or ulcers can be treated. Research in the USA has indicated that the eclectic approach can be an effective alternative to antibiotics, antivirals and surgery for some chronic conditions (Pizzorno & Murray 1999).

Bearing in mind the philosophy of naturopathy, irrespective of the therapies used by practitioners, the patient will be treated as a unique individual. Case history taking will encompass all aspects of the holistic approach, so that the physical, biochemical, environmental, hereditary and psychological aspects of the individual are considered. Questions will therefore include general health including musculoskeletal aches and pains, diet and bowel habits, home and work environment, childhood illnesses and family history, alcohol and tobacco intake, stressors and the patients' psychological condition.

Therapeutic potential in nursing

Nurses trained in naturopathy would have many skills to offer as members of a health care team. For example, homeopathy has much to offer in community care, midwifery and day nursing. See the chapter on homeopathy (chapter 23) for details of how it may be useful in Accident and Emergency Department, Intensive Care and medical and surgical units, provided the necessary authorization is obtained. In addition research has indicated that massage may have considerable therapeutic potential in nursing for example in the reduction of anxiety (Fraser & Ross Kerr 1993) and in improved lymphatic circulation (Morgan et al 1992). Many of the underpinning approaches and therapies used by naturopaths have therapeutic potential in nursing. However, it is probably the philosophical approach which has much in common with good nursing practice that has most therapeutic potential.

Contraindications for use

The safety, effectiveness and cost-effectiveness of naturopathic medicine has been well documented (Pizzorno & Murray 1999). Due to the philosophical approach of natural medicine being used to support and stimulate the healing power of nature, therapies are used only after careful consideration of the patient's needs as an individual. The contraindications of specific therapies used by naturopaths are detailed in the respective chapters of this book. However, it is important to remember that an accepted aspect of naturopathic treatment is the support and stimulation of the body's attempts to eliminate unwanted or toxic materials through fevers, mild aches and pains, sweating, swellings and in some cases diarrhoea or vomiting. These responses, which are referred to by naturopaths as symptoms of a 'healing crisis', should not be suppressed as they are an indication of the body's attempt to regain homeostasis or balance.

Summary

Naturopathy is an approach to health care founded on the belief that the body has the power to heal itself. The multidisciplinary approach using gentle or natural therapies may, however, appear to be slow in achieving a therapeutic response. In naturopathy the attempts of the body to eliminate materials must not be suppressed, therefore some symptoms may be experienced during the healing process. Some of the therapies used by naturopaths involve touch which is an integral part of nursing care. The use of massage or bodywork can make a valuable contribution in providing a relaxing and caring environment. However, it is probably the philosophical approach, particularly the four basic principles shared with good nursing practice, that are likely to make the most significant contribution to the therapeutic potential of naturopathy.

This information will contribute to the practitioner's decision regarding which therapies to use. Routine assessments usually carried out include temperature, respiratory rate, pulse, blood pressure and weight; laboratory tests may be performed as well if necessary.

CURRENT RESEARCH

Most of the research into the effectiveness of naturopathic medicine has been undertaken at Bastyr University in the USA. The results of early research have been recorded in the *Textbook of Natural Medicine* by Pizzorno & Murray (1999). Studies into ear infections in children have indicated that naturopathy was an effective alternative to antibiotics and surgery. The results of a study of HIV-positive patients treated for a year with hydrotherapy, homeopathy, herbal remedies and supplementation revealed 75% reported improved well-being and none of the group developed AIDS. However, as with all complementary therapies it is imperative that further research is carried to evaluate their effectiveness.

REFERENCES

Featherstone C Forsyth L 1997 Medical marriage, the new partnership between orthodox and complementary medicine. Findhorn Press, Scotland
Fraser J Ross Kerr J 1993 Psychophysiological effects of back massage in elderly institutionalised patients. Journal of Advanced Nursing 18: 238–245
Micozzi M S 1996 Fundamentals of complementary and alternative medicine. Churchill Livingstone, New York
Morgan R G et al 1992 Complex physical therapy for the lymphoedematous arm. Journal of Hand Surgery 178: 437–441
Peters D Lewis P J Chaitow L Watson C 1996 Chronic fatigue. Complementary Therapies in Medicine 4: 31–38
Pizzorno J E Murray M T 1999 Textbook of natural medicine, 2nd edn. Churchill Livingstone, London, vols I and II
Woodham A Peters D 1997 Encyclopedia of complementary medicine. Dorling Kindersley, London

FURTHER READING – BOOKS

Chaitow L 1995 Stress. Thorsons, London
Chaitow L 1996 Principles of fasting. Thorsons, London
Chaitow L 1999 Hydrotherapy. Element, England
Davies N Harrold F 1990 Massage cures. Thorsons, London
Lindlahr H 1975 Philosophy of natural therapeutics. C W Daniel, London
Millenson J 1996 Mind matters – psychological medicine in holistic practice. Eastland, USA

USEFUL ADDRESSES

British College of Naturopathy & Osteopathy
Lief House
3 Sumpter Close
120–122 Finchley Road
London NW3 5HR
Tel: 020 7435 6464

Centre for Community Care & Primary Health
University of Westminster

115 New Cavendish Street
London W1M 8JS
Tel: 020 7911 5082

The British Naturopathic Association
Goswell House
2 Goswell Road
Street
Somerset BA16 0JG
Tel: 01458 840 072

29 Osteopathy

Brian Daniels

Osteopathy – *the BMA's 1993 Report on Complementary Medicine (British Medical Association, Complementary Medicine, New Approaches to Good Practice, 1993) describes osteopathy as a 'discrete clinical discipline'. It is, in fact, an established system of assessment (the patient being assessed from a mechanical, functional and postural standpoint), clinical diagnosis and manual treatment. A caring approach and attention paid to individual needs are fundamental.*

In particular, osteopathy is concerned with the inter-relationship between the structure of the body and the way the body functions and it is, therefore, an appropriate therapeutic approach to many problems affecting the neuro-musculo-skeletal systems.

Well-known as an effective treatment for back pain, in fact osteopaths use a wide variety of approaches, including the cranial and visceral approaches, and can bring relief or improvement to many conditions. These range from problems that arise during and after pregnancy and conditions affecting children such as 'glue ear' to digestive and intestinal problems and respiratory disorders such as asthma (the osteopath working to improve the way in which muscles control breathing and to reduce joint restrictions and stiffness).

The profession of osteopathy in the UK is currently undergoing major change. The passage of the Osteopaths Act 1993 was the successful conclusion of a 70-year campaign by osteopaths. The establishment under the Act of the General Osteopathic Council (GOsC) meant that osteopathy became the first of the professions complementary to medicine to achieve statutory self-regulation on a similar model to that of the doctors and dentists.

The GOsC exists to protect patients by promoting excellence in osteopathic care by:

- maintaining a statutory register
- promoting high standards of osteopathic education

- guiding osteopaths in standards of professional practice. The GOsC has published a code of practice (General Osteopathic Council, Pursuing Excellence, June 1998) that states clearly the standards expected of a Registered Osteopath
- acting when an osteopath's fitness to practice is questioned
- promoting and developing the practice of osteopathy.

Central to the legislation is protection of the title 'osteopath' (or derivatives of it). Only those practitioners who gain admittance to the GOsC's statutory register, currently by completing a rigorous evaluation process and, after May 2000, by graduating with a recognized qualification from an accredited institution, will be able to call themselves osteopaths.

In addition to bringing important safeguards for the public, statutory regulation is also serving to enhance professional relationships within health care and to open new opportunities. Changes to GMC guidelines (General Medical Council, Guideline for Good Medical Practice, 38–42, July 1998), for example, make it clear that doctors may refer patients to osteopaths for investigation, care or treatment which falls outside the doctor's competence. Even more significantly, specialists such as radiologists and orthopaedic surgeons may now accept patients referred directly by a Registered Osteopath without another doctor having to act as an intermediary.

A recent survey (General Osteopathic Council, Osteopathy 'Snapshot' Survey, February 1998) revealed that over a quarter of patients attended an osteopath with their doctors' approval, over 10% being formally referred. In addition, a national survey (Anglo European College of Chiropractic, British School of Osteopathy, Southampton University Physiotherapy Department, Unpublished Research Collaboration, 1999) found almost 400 osteopaths in the UK who had at some time undertaken NHS work (mainly as independent practitioners contracted to a fundholding General Practice).

HISTORICAL BACKGROUND

Osteopathy emerged as a system of manual medicine in the USA in the 1870s, challenging the dependence of contemporary orthodox medical practice on drugs and surgery. Its pioneer, Dr Andrew Taylor Still, founded osteopathy on two basic principles that remain valid today. The first is that the body contains within itself the means to combat disease and maintain health. The second is that structure and function are inter-related and, if the structure of the body is sound, the body is better able to function well and maintain health or recover from disease.

Osteopathic medicine was introduced into England in 1898 when Dr John Martin Littlejohn, a Glaswegian physiologist who had trained with Still, gave a paper at the Society of Science, Letters and Arts entitled 'Osteopathy – in line of apostolic succession to medicine'. In 1917, Littlejohn established Europe's first osteopathic school, the British School of Osteopathy, in London. From these early beginnings, today the UK's 2500 osteopaths give over six million patient consultations a year.

Training

Currently in the UK, there is a choice of several modes of educational process, from 4-year, full-time courses to 5-year extended pathway and part-time courses, most now leading to a BSc degree. There is also a 13-month course for the postgraduate training of registered medical practitioners. Undergraduate training includes a thorough knowledge of the basic medical sciences, together with extensive clinical training that is central to the osteopath's ability to make a differential diagnosis and to distinguish relative and absolute contraindications to manual treatment.

Currently, the GOsC has begun the task of assessing osteopathic institutions, those accredited being enabled to award a 'recognized qualification', the major requirement for statutory registration after May 2000. Central to the process is for the institutions to demonstrate that the requirements of a new standard of proficiency (General Osteopathic Council, Standard 2000, March 1999) are being met.

TREATMENT

The osteopath's approach to diagnosis and treatment (taking a typical patient presenting with low back pain as the example) is as follows:

Patient's history

Patients are taken through a detailed history of their current problem, including time and mode of onset, extent, duration and severity of previous episodes and prior investigations and treatment. When related to patient age, this should categorize suspicions into congenital, developmental, traumatic, degenerative or pathological areas.

Thorough exploration of the factors that aggravate or relieve the condition reveals the extent of daily dysfunction and the patient's expectations of function. It also determines whether this dysfunction is of mechanical origin or whether pathological or psychosocial elements should be questioned. Past medical history of illness, operations, investigations and treatment, as well as enquiry into current systemic health, is necessary. The history invariably produces a diagnostic hypothesis to be confirmed or refuted by examination.

It is important to note that because the majority of presenting symptoms are mechanical in origin, osteopaths are diligent in identifying those that are not.

Examination

Observing the standing patient reveals information about physique as well as the antero-posterior and lateral plane postural balance. Skin folds and muscle hyper/hypo-tonicity are identified. Pelvic balance is examined before undertaking and recording full active movement. Sitting examination is routine to establish alterations in pelvic balance and the effect of the lumbar spine falling into flexion. The recumbent patient may undergo assessment of leg lengths.

Passive palpatory examination is one of the hallmarks of osteopathy, from which a full segmental analysis is constructed and related to the patient's weight-bearing posture. Ranges of individual segments are recorded and intrinsic and extrinsic soft tissue assessed. Neurological and other systemic examinations are undertaken at this stage. If X-rays are required for structural information, which may define structural expectations, these will be arranged.

The osteopath will now have constructed a complete evaluation of the patient's spinal function and the factors that collectively caused the symptoms. Emphasis is placed on identifying postural, occupational or habitual factors that may be maintaining the problem. A treatment plan, including lifestyle and postural advice and exercise is constructed for the patient as an individual. Standardization of diagnostic groups and treatment regimes does not work well in the osteopathic setting where a multiplicity of factors identifies patients as individuals.

Diagnosis

Osteopaths do not treat conditions per se. They evaluate and treat patients holistically. For example, someone presenting with low back pain could have a problem with foot mechanics. Their evaluative model has many facets in terms of musculoskeletal, emotional and lifestyle factors. To give a list of individual afflictions that may be amenable or are contraindicated would be misleading and would tend to limit the scope of practice.

Osteopaths take responsibility for their own diagnosis. They are trained to recognize contraindications to treatment and will refer as appropriate.

Treatment

Osteopaths work with their hands using a wide variety of treatment techniques. These may include soft tissue stretching techniques, rhythmic passive movements to improve joint mobility or high velocity thrust techniques designed to improve the mobility and range of movement of a joint (the audible click).

The current understanding of the biopsychosocial concept in relation to structural dysfunction and the relevance to therapeutic planning has long been part of osteopathic health care. Osteopaths monitor progress in relation to the negotiated expectations of practitioner and patient. The patient is encouraged to understand and share in the treatment, which is one important element in creating an effective clinical outcome. Continual critical reflection of progress and fine-tuning of management is paramount. If results fall short, a review of diagnosis and treatment is undertaken. Communication and discussion with the patient's GP may be necessary.

The amount of treatment a patient will require is dependent upon their individual characteristics and it is now recognized that structural characteristics are more often than not related to genetic factors. The osteopath's assessment skills come to the fore in determining appropriate therapeutic approaches that are focused on each individual

Therapeutic potential in nursing

Research results offer encouraging indications. There are many publications from around the world that report trials and evaluations for musculoskeletal problems, especially low back pain. Findings and conclusions generally relate to the effectiveness of spinal manipulation or manipulative therapies in general, rather than stand-alone findings on osteopathy.

Koes et al (1996) found that 'there certainly are indications that manipulation might be effective in some sub-groups of patients with low back pain'.

Similarly, Assendelft et al (1995) found that 'nine out of the ten methodologically best reviews were positive' (in terms of the effectiveness of spinal manipulation for low back pain). Their conclusion stated that 'The majority of the reviews concluded that spinal manipulation is an effective treatment for low back pain'.

Another recent review (van Tulder et al 1997) reports 'strong evidence for the effectiveness of manipulation for chronic low back pain, especially for short-term effects'.

At present, there is a large-scale, randomized clinical trial of low back pain treatment taking place in the UK (funded by the MRC) that includes osteopathy. The UK BEAM Trial, as it is known, will not produce and publish findings until 2002–2004.

patient, acknowledging each patient's limitations but with diference to their expectations.

An average for acute back pain of between four and six treatments appears to be the norm.

Summary

Experience within the NHS arena suggests that major benefits are:

- the osteopath's clinical assessment skills reduce the risk of illness behaviour by avoiding unnecessary diagnostic investigations, imaging and consultant referral
- osteopathy can reduce the amount of NSAIDs prescribed
- a reduction in repeat visits to a GP frees GP appointment time
- early osteopathic intervention achieves early relief of symptoms.

REFERENCES

Assendelft W J Koes B W Knipschild P G Bouter L M 1995 The relationship between methodological quality and conclusions in reviews of spinal manipulation. JAMA 274 (24): 1942–1948

Koes B W Assendelft W J van der Heijden G L Bouter L M 1996 Spinal manipulation for low back pain. An updated systematic review of randomised clinical trials. Spine 21 (24): 2860–2871

Van Tulder M W Koes B W Bouter L M 1997 Conservative treatment of acute and chronic non-specific low back pain. A systematic review of randomised controlled trials of the most common interventions. Spine 22 (18): 2128–2156

USEFUL ADDRESS

General Osteopathic Council
Osteopathy House
176 Tower Bridge Road
London SE1 3LU
Tel: 020 7357 6655

30 Reflexology

Pamela Griffiths

Reflexology – *a treatment which applies varying degrees of pressure to different parts of the body, usually the hands or feet, in order to promote health and well-being.*

The term 'reflexology' to some extent describes the basis of this therapy. It is suggested that there are reflexes or zones running along the body which terminate in the hands or feet. All systems and organs of the body are said to be reflected on to the surface of the skin, in particular on to the hands and feet. Thus, by applying gentle pressure to these areas it is possible to effect a change in another part of the body in order to promote well-being and relaxation. This form of therapy can influence not only specific organs but also the relationship between organs, other systems and processes (Goodwin 1988).

Depending upon the type of training undertaken by a practitioner one of several techniques may be adopted during therapy. However, the underlying principles of the different methods are consistent. Methods may include:

- Traditional reflexology – Bailey, Ingham (Hall 1986)
- Reflex zone therapy (Marquardt 1983)
- Metamorphic technique (Saint-Pierre & Shapiro 1989)
- Morrell method (Hewetson 1989)
- Holistic multidimensional reflexology (Ashkenazi 1993)
- Vacuflex reflexology (Dougans and Ellis 1982)

Botting (1997) suggests that reflexology may be used to treat a variety of conditions, particularly those of a chronic nature such as pain in arthritis or sciatica, back pain and gastrointestinal tract disturbances, skin problems and menstrual problems (Barron 1990, Booth 1994). It can also encourage self-healing (Shaw 1987, Sahai 1993). Cromwell et al (1999) have written about the concept of a 'healing crisis' which may occur during treatment. Tiran (1996) has described the use of reflexology in midwifery practice. Definitions of reflexology also vary (see Box).

A sample of definitions of reflexology

'Reflexology is a method for stimulating the reflexes in the feet to cause reactions in corresponding parts of the body. The reaction could best be described as relaxation, or a return to equilibrium' Kunz & Kunz (1984).

'The foot is assumed to contain a reflex area that corresponds to every organ and every part of the body ... Reflexologists believe that by treating the reflex area with pressure, they can clear energy blockages' Frydenlund (1992).

'...reflexology refers to a method of treatment whereby reflex points in the feet are massaged in a particular way to bring about an effect in areas of the body quite distant from the feet' Hall (1986).

'Reflexology is a method for activating the healing powers of the body ... reflexology works with subtle energy flows, revitalizing the body so that the natural internal healing mechanisms of the body can do their own work' Norman (1989).

'Reflexology is a therapy based on a belief that the body's natural healing mechanisms can be enhanced by the application of pressure to certain areas of the feet and hands. These areas are said to be connected to different parts of the body by a flow of energy. The term reflex refers to the "reflection" of organs on the skin's surface, hence the name "reflexology"' Booth (1993).

There is a vast amount of anecdotal evidence claiming support for reflexology (Wynn 1988, Evans 1990). However, there is a need for validating therapies scientifically (Mercer et al 1995). There are an increasing number of scientific studies being undertaken in this field (Lafuente et al 1990, Kovaks et al 1993, Olsen & Flocco 1993, Wang 1993, Frankel 1997). Few large-scale research studies have been undertaken addressing the effectiveness of reflexology.

HISTORICAL BACKGROUND

There is evidence to suggest that the therapeutic use of hand and foot pressure for the treatments of pain and various illnesses was in existence in China and India over 5000 years ago and it was also used by American Indian tribes (Goodwin 1988). A wall painting in the Egyptian tomb of Ankhmahor Saqqara 2300 BC depicts this therapy.

More recent descriptions of reflexology are commonly attributed to studies at the end of the nineteenth century by Dr William Fitzgerald, an American ear, nose and throat specialist. Fitzgerald found, quite by accident, that gentle pressure applied to specific parts of the hand or foot could cause partial local anaesthesia in areas of the ear, nose and throat. By using pressure points on the hands and feet, Fitzgerald claimed to be able to perform minor surgery without conventional anaesthetics (Goodwin 1988).

Fitzgerald attempted to map the areas or zones of the hands and feet and, in 1917, in association with Dr Edwin Bowers published a treatise describing reflex zone therapy (Berkson 1977). This identified ten zones running through the body and gave maps of the internal organs reflected on the hands and feet. Fitzgerald suggested that controlled pressure with the fingers and thumbs at the end of these zones could produce a response elsewhere in the body. He claimed that reflexology stimulated not only the organ but also the interrelationship between organs and other body systems.

In 1920, Riley further developed this method and his book *Zone Therapy Simplified* describes horizontal zones of the feet (Marquardt 1983, Goodwin 1988). More recently, Eunice Ingham, a research assistant with Riley, refined this theory and attempted to define precise zone pathways. Ingham maintains that by focusing on foot pressure, all parts of the body may be treated (Booth 1993). In the early 1960s, Doreen Bailey met Ingham whilst in America and upon her return to the UK, began to practise and encourage interest in reflexology here.

The concept of channels of energy flowing around the body is not unique to reflexology; therapeutic touch, acupuncture and shiatsu are based on similar theories of an innate body energy that can be treated on the body surface to stimulate internal organs. Dougans & Ellis (1992) suggest that reflexology, like acupuncture, works with the meridians but much more research on these 'energy pathways' is needed.

TREATMENT

Reflexology suggests that every part of the body is connected by reflex zones or pathways terminating in the soles of the feet, palms of the hands, ears, tongue and head (Corvo 1990, Ashkenazi 1993). The reflex zones relate to all areas of the body through ten longitudinal zones, which are symmetrical, with five on each side of the body.

Tension, congestion or some other imbalance will affect the whole zone and it is possible to treat one part of the zone, such as the foot, to bring about a change in other specified parts of the body (Barron 1990). Ingham considered that malfunction of any organ or part of the body resulted in tiny crystalline deposits of calcium and uric acid on the nerve endings of the feet (Goodwin 1988). Gentle pressure is thought to facilitate the breakdown and elimination of these deposits and so promote health and well-being (Ingham 1938). This is referred to as detoxification and the signs that it is occurring as a 'healing crisis'. Once this process has occurred, healing can begin.

The foot is treated by applying gentle pressure along each zone systematically until the entire foot has been covered. This includes the dorsum, sides and top – then the same process is carried out on the other foot. Initially, gentle massage and stroking movements are used, followed by deep thumb and finger pressures. If there is an imbalance or blockage of energy in any of the zones or reflexes, they may feel tender or painful and gentle pressures are applied to remove the blockage. Reflex treatment is said to treat the body on a number of levels simultaneously: the sole of the foot has areas relating to specific organs and also to the emotions. The treatment can influence emotional, physical and spiritual disorders (Goodwin 1988).

After treatment, a healing crisis may occur due to detoxification of the body (Sahai 1993). Some examples of healing crisis symptoms are as follows:

- 'Flu-like' symptoms
- Feeling light-headed, very relaxed
- Feeling very cold 3–4 days post-treatment
- Increase in excretory functions
- Reduction in blood pressure
- Lethargy
- Enhanced or altered sleep pattern.

It is essential that nurses are aware of and able to manage symptoms of a reflexology healing crisis, as distinct from pathological conditions, and know when to refer to other health care practitioners. Thus, a good training course is recommended before using reflexology in professional practice.

Training in reflexology

This technique may be harmful if not used correctly, despite the popular belief that it is a simple foot massage. There is no current governing body for training and there are several schools with varying course length, student numbers and standards. Courses should be a minimum of one year, and preferably affiliated to a professional body such as the British Register of Health Practitioners or the Association of Reflexologists (AOR). The AOR, founded in 1984, aims to monitor and maintain standards of professional practice. Nurses can also consult the Royal College of Nursing Special Interest Group Guidelines on Complementary Therapy Courses (RCNSIG 1993).

There are educational programmes in reflexology accredited by the ENB and universities, some offering courses at levels 2 and 3. It would also be useful to refer here to the FIM recommendations on education and regulation. The Reflexology Organisations Council has recently been established to help the development of standards and representation of reflexology at a national level (FIM 1997).

Types of treatment

Some of the techniques based on traditional zone therapy are outlined next.

Holistic reflexology

Morrell and holistic multidimensional reflexology treatments last about 30 minutes and use the same zone theory but mirror image each move from foot to foot, rather than zone to zone, using ultragentle palpation of the feet. Alterations in skin tone and texture are identified and all imbalances of the feet are painlessly treated with minimum healing crisis reaction. This is due to the resultant deep relaxation; respiratory rate, pulse and heart rate are decreased, blood pressure is homeostatically balanced, and stimulation of healing energies is achieved (Dougans & Ellis 1992). Owing to these physiological changes, homeostasis can be regained and maintained. This results in relief of symptoms, and facilitates the rebuilding and rebalancing of energies required to aid healing and prevent illness. The author, whilst taking part in a pilot study on orthopaedic patients, found that after treatment most patients were more relaxed, in less pain and able to sleep better.

Metamorphic technique

This approach was developed by Robert St John in the 1960s, working on the theory that the foot mirrors the 9-month gestation period in utero and that problems that develop in utero go on to later life. Early therapy may remove the problems. The feet, hands and head are gently rubbed to relieve the pressure said to be causing blockages in energy flow (Gonzales & Saint-Pierre 1992).

Vacuflex reflexology

This is a two-phase treatment linking reflex stimulation and meridian rebalancing. Specially developed suction boots are put on the feet and suction cups in specific areas of the body stimulate the reflexes, when connected to a suction pump. The theory combines reflexology, acupressure and cupping to bring about homeostasis (Dougans & Ellis 1992).

Therapeutic potential in nursing

Reflexology offers a wide range of potential benefits for nurses practising within a multidisciplinary team in all health sectors. Maternity and care of the elderly are showing particular interest in this therapy. Many conditions and ages may be treated by qualified therapists. Most conditions respond within a few sessions, depending on the individual. Note, however, that not everyone will find the intensity of the treatment acceptable. Therapeutic benefits include:

- Pain relief in acute and chronic states
- Control of anxiety
- Reduction in blood pressure, pulse, temperature and hormone levels, thereby improving circulation, breathing and elimination
- Deep relaxation
- Relief of tension in Alzheimer's disease
- Relief of glue ear (paediatrics)
- Skin healing (diabetes)
- Relaxation in pregnancy/birth
- Detoxification
- Revitalizing and rebalancing effects, facilitating healing
- Immune system strengthening
- Improved (rapid eye movement) sleep
- Preventive measure as part of health promotion
- Wound healing – varicose ulcers.

Treatment should only be carried out by a trained practitioner and preferably as part of a multidisciplinary approach. Cross-professional referring of clients ensures the most effective system of care.

Contraindications for use

- Some individuals may find the intensity of this therapy unacceptable.
- It is not generally used for diagnosis, except in preventive health care (Morrell or holistic multidimensional reflexology).
- For some conditions, e.g. diabetes and hyper/hypothyroidism, the reflexologist must work closely with medical colleagues.
- Traditional reflexology is not suitable for the first trimester of pregnancy.
- It should be used cautiously with patients in depressive and manic states.
- Use with care in epilepsy and in acute conditions.

Summary

Reflexology is potentially a very valuable therapeutic nursing skill and could have wide-ranging and cost-effective benefits in health care, from special care baby units through to care of the elderly. Like many other complementary therapies, reflexology seems to restore and maintain health by rebalancing the body. Whilst to many, reflexology may appear a gentle therapy, it is vital that the contraindications are known and that it is only carried out by trained therapists.

REFERENCES

Ashkenazi R 1993 Multidimensional reflexology. International Journal of Alternative and Complementary Medicine June: 8–12

Barron H 1990 Towards better health with reflexology. Nursing Standard 4: 32–33

Berkson D 1977 The foot book – healing the body through reflexology. Barnes & Nobles, New York

Booth B 1993 Complementary therapy. Nursing Times/Macmillan, London

Booth B 1994 Reflexology. Nursing Times 5: 38–40

Botting D 1997 Review of the literature on the effectiveness of reflexology. Complementary Therapies in Nursing & Midwifery. 3: 125–130

Corvo J 1990 Zone therapy. Century, London

Cromwell C Dryden S Jones D Mackereth P 1999 'Just the ticket'; case studies, reflections and clinical supervision (Part III). Complementary Therapies in Nursing & Midwifery 5: 42–45

Dougans I Ellis S 1992 The art of reflexology. Element, Dorset

Evans M 1990 Reflex zone therapy for mothers. Nursing Times 86 (4): 29–32

FIM (Foundation For Integrated Medicine) 1997 Integrated Healthcare: a way forward for the next five years? FIM, London

Frankel B 1997 The effects of reflexology on baroreceptors reflex sensitivity, blood pressure and sinus arrhythmia. Complementary Therapies in Medicine 5: 80–84

Frydenlund J 1992 Reflexology – a training book. Spottrup, Denmark

Gonzales M A Saint-Pierre G 1992 Any difference between reflexology and the metamorphic technique? Metamorphosis 26: 69–71

Goodwin H 1988 Reflex zone therapy cited in Rankin-Box D (ed) Complementary health therapies: a guide for nurses and the caring professions. Chapman and Hall, London

Griffiths P 1993 Tickling innovation in Cardiff. Full House Conference Report Orthopaedic Bare Bone No 20 Autumn newsletter. Society of Orthopaedic Nursing, Royal College of Nursing. Smith and Nephew, London

Hall N M 1986 Reflexology: a patients guide. Thorsons, Wellingborough

Hewetson R 1989 Feet first. Haps (Chepstow), Bristol

Ingham E 1938 Stories the feet can tell. Ingham, St Petersburg, Florida

Kovaks F M Abraira V Lopez-Abente G Pozo F 1993 Neuro-reflexology intervention in the treatment of non-specified low back pain. In: Association of Reflexologists (1994) Reflexology Research Reports (2nd edn) A.O.R. London

Kunz K Kunz B 1984 The complete Guide to foot reflexology. Thorsons, London

Lafuente A Noquera M Puy C Molins A Titus F Sanz F 1990 Effekt der Reflexzonenbehandlung an Fuss bezüglich der prophylaktischen Behandlung mit Flunarizin bei einen Cephalea–Kopfschmerzen leidenden Patienten. Erfahrungscheilkunde 39 (11): 713–715

Mackereth P A 1999 An introduction to catharsis and the healing crisis in reflexology. Complementary Therapies in Nursing & Midwifery, 5: 67–74

Marquardt H 1983 Reflex zone therapy of the feet. Thorsons, Wellingborough

Mercer G Long A F Smith I J 1995 Researching and evaluating complementary therapies: the state of the debate. Nuffield Institute for Health, University of Leeds

Norman L 1989 The reflexology handbook – a complete guide. Piatkus, London

Oleson J Flocco W 1993 Randomised controlled study of premenstrual symptoms treated with ear, hand and foot reflexology. Obstetrics & Gynaecology 82 (6): 906–911

Sahai I C M 1993 Reflexology – its place in modern health care. Professional Nurse 18: 722–725

Shaw J 1987 Reflexology. Health Visitor 60 (11): 367

Tiran D 1996 The use of complementary therapies in midwifery practice: a focus on reflexology. Complementary Therapies in Nursing & Midwifery, 2: 32–37

Wang X M 1993 Treating Type II diabetes mellitus with foot reflextherapy. Chung–Kuo Chung Hsi i Chieh Ho Tsa Chin 13 (9): 536–538

Wynn S 1988 Reflex Zone Therapy. Nursing Standard 2 (17): 28

FURTHER READING

Bayley D E 1982 Reflexology today (revised edn). Thorsons, Wellingborough

Dryden S Holden S Mackereth P 1998 'Just the ticket'; integrating massage and reflexology in practice (Part I). Complementary Therapies in Nursing & Midwifery 4: 154–159

Dryden S Holden S Mackereth P 1999 'Just the ticket'; the findings of a pilot complementary therapy service (Part II). Complementary Therapies in Nursing & Midwifery 5: 15–18

Joyce M Richardson R 1997 Reflexology can help MS. International Journal of Alternative and Complementary Medicine July Edition: 10–12

Kunz K Kunz B 1986 Hand and foot reflexology. Thorsons, Wellingborough

Norman L Cowan T 1989 The reflexology handbook. Piatkus, London

Richards W J 1990 Sole searching. Here's Health 34: 37

Trousdall P 1996 Reflexology meets emotional needs. International Journal of Alternative and Complementary Medicine. November Edition: 9–12

USEFUL ADDRESSES

Association of Reflexologists
27 Old Gloucester Street
London WC1 3XX
Tel: 020 7237 6523

Association of Vacuflex
Reflexologists
25 Meadowcroft Close
East Grinstead, West Sussex
RNH19 1NA,
Tel: 01342 24019

British Reflexology Association
Monks Orchard,
Whitbourne
Worcester WR6 5RB
Tel: 01886 212707

British School – Reflex Zone
Therapy of the Feet
87 Oakington Avenue
Wembley Park
London HA9 8HY
Tel: 020 8908 2201

Holistic Association of British
Reflexologists
92 Sheering Road
Old Harrow
Essex CM17 0JW
Tel: 01279 429060

Metamorphic Association
67 Ritherdon Road
London SW17 8QE
Tel: 020 8672 5951

31 Relaxation and visualization

Lynne Ryman   Denise Rankin-Box

Relaxation – *a state of consciousness characterized by feelings of peace and release from tension, anxiety and fear.*

Visualization – *using the imagination to create desired changes in an individual's life.*

Relaxation and visualization are planned and structured activities leading to peace of mind and enhanced quality of life (Ryman 1994). In this respect, successful practice of relaxation and visualization techniques can result in the ability to control and reduce tension, worry and anxiety (Ryman 1994). It is increasingly well-accepted and documented that excessive stress interferes with a person's well-being and ability to enjoy life (Friedman et al 1969, Selye 1976). Where tension is experienced over long periods of time this may have a depressing effect on the immune system leading to ill-health and disease (Ryman 1994). For total health and happiness all aspects of human experience, emotional, physical, mental, psychological and spiritual, need to be in a balanced state and in harmony with each other; disease can occur when they are not (Simonton et al 1978).

Relaxation and visualization work together to provide a therapy which encourages negative unhealthy states of mind to be replaced by positive healthy ones. The role of relaxation is to bring the mind of the participant to a state of balance and peace. Visualization uses this balanced state to remove negative or self-destructive thoughts and move towards a better state, as perceived by the client. Relaxation and visualization can facilitate health-giving changes, and promote reduction in the physical and mental effects of stress, encouraging therapeutic benefits such as reduced blood pressure and lower levels of stress hormones (Woodham & Peters 1997).

Relaxation and visualization provide a necessary and healing break in the daily routine; they are strategies for self-healing and illness prevention when used regularly. Relaxation of body, mind and spirit is one way in which to regain and maintain a healthy, harmonious, whole human being (Ryman 1994).

HISTORICAL BACKGROUND

The many ways in which people can learn to reduce levels of stress are well documented. Throughout history peace of mind has been gained by repetitive praying (teaching the mind to dwell on one thought) and by meditation (Benson & Klipper 1977). One of the first modern techniques developed for stress reduction was 'progressive relaxation' (Jacobson 1977), based on the idea that muscle tension or relaxation influences the state of the entire person. In progressive relaxation, the person tenses and then relaxes successive groups of muscles, focusing attention on the differences experienced when muscles are in a tense or relaxed state (Ryman 1994). Jacobson's technique entailed learning to relax 218 different muscle groups and required perseverance and time to master successfully.

The relaxation response devised by Benson in 1974 is a simpler process that almost anyone can use. It requires the following:

- A quiet environment
- A word or phrase repeated over and over again
- The adoption of a passive attitude
- A comfortable position.

Regular practice should promote a markedly enhanced state of well-being (Benson & Klipper 1977, Ryman 1994). At first Benson felt that the four basic components listed were essential. Subsequently he specified just two:

- Repetition of a word, a sound, a prayer, a phrase or a muscular movement
- Passive disregard of everyday thoughts when they occur.

Other techniques used to achieve a relaxed state include autogenic training, biofeedback, hypnosis and slow stroke massage, to mention but a few.

Visualization is the use of mental imaging to alleviate and prevent disease. This practice has been documented throughout history and is commonly associated with American and African shamanism. Some oriental therapies also made use of visualization (Reader's Digest 1991, Ryman 1994). Since the early 1970s the names of Carl and Stephanie Simonton (Simonton 1978) have become synonymous with visualization following their extensive use of this method in working with severe illness, such as cancer. The subject is taught to focus on an appropriate image, preferably of their choice, to induce a feeling of peace or happiness or to promote beneficial changes in health or circumstance.

Relaxation and visualization methods are being increasingly researched world-wide, to discover whether and how states of mind can influence physiological changes in the body and psychological well-being (Meares 1979, Patel et al 1985, Chang 1991).

TREATMENT

Everyone has an innate self-protective mechanism against too much stress. This 'relaxation response' (Benson & Klipper 1977) is characterized by decreased heart rate, lowered metabolism, decreased rate of breathing and slower brain waves, which help return the body to a healthier balanced state.

As part of a structured programme to promote health-giving, deep breathing and progressive muscle relaxation techniques can be used on their own or for greater benefit in combination with visualization. The basic technique (Ryman 1994) is outlined next.

Participants sit comfortably with eyes closed, feet firmly fixed on the floor, spine supported and fingers and feet uncrossed. The session usually lasts for 30 to 45 minutes and the theme of self-awareness and seeing oneself in one's mind's eye is encouraged throughout. There are generally three parts to the session in the following order:

- Observation of the normal breathing pattern, its rate, rhythm and depth, followed by deeper breathing.
- Progressive muscle relaxation – tensing and relaxing major muscle groups throughout the body paying particular attention to sensing the opposite poles of tension and relaxation.
- The visualization exercise, in which participants are first encouraged to experience, for example, a country walk with all their senses (sight, touch, smell, taste, hearing). From the peaceful state achieved by this, they move on to more specific visualizations designed to address current issues, for example:
  — a war waged between good cells and diseased cells (with the good cells winning)
  — picturing a laser beam destroying tissue affected by disease (and leaving good tissue free)
  — seeing in every detail a desired scenario, such as being full of well-being, wholeness and happiness
  — an improved relationship
  — being free of pain.

Researchers now believe that the images used in the visualization above should be chosen by the individuals themselves, since they are more likely to be relevant and therefore effective (Simonton 1978). Good images are subjective and unique, in line with the individualistic approach of many complementary therapies.

It is very important that on completion of the exercise each participant is well grounded before resuming normal activity. Regular practice is necessary, since a cumulative effect gives the best results. Tapes for home use are helpful.

Stages of technique

Stage I
— normal level of consciousness
— full awareness
— beta brain wave, characterized by decision-making, reasoning and logic
— emotions: full range

Stage II
— changed level of consciousness
— relaxed mellowness
— alpha brain wave, characterized by a lessening effect of negative thoughts and feelings
— emotions: stilled, muted

Stage III
— changed level of consciousness
— very lucid: intense alertness
— alpha/theta or alpha/beta, characterized by openness to ideas of creativity, inspiration and healing
— emotions; calmness and detachment; deeply satisfying

Therapeutic potential in nursing

A growing number of hospitals now offer on a regular basis relaxation and visualization to their staff and patients in the form of self-help groups. Below are some of the benefits:

■ Hypertension: a non-pharmacological way of reducing high blood pressure (mild, acute and chronic)

■ Insomnia: aids return to a normal sleep pattern, leading to reaffirmation of homeostasis

■ Coronary artery disease: provides a way for reversing heart disease without the use of drugs or surgery

■ Arthritis: lessens pain/disabilities; aids regression of disease

■ Stress management: reduces levels of tension, anxiety and stress, leading to a more balanced outlook on life

■ Potentially painful procedures: through self-awareness and self-control decreases distress and discomfort without sedation

■ Immune system: strengthens to give less susceptibility to disease

Therapeutic potential in nursing (cont'd)

- Pain, management of all forms: reduction with relaxation alone but increased efficiency when used with visualization
- Positive outlook: lessens negativity and renews hope; allows clients to take part in their own healing
- Reduction in side effects such as nausea and vomiting caused by radiotherapy, chemotherapy; decreased analgesia postoperatively
- Cancer: can help to reduce anger, anxiety and depression caused by trauma of disease
- Relaxation: facilitates peace of mind and insight into the nature of one's problems and the influence of attitude in dealing with these issues
- Coping mechanisms: increases ability to cope, re-energizes, leads to an improvement in quality of life
- Panic attacks: can reduce fear and lead to reduction of symptoms and an understanding of the cause of anxiety.

Contraindications for use

- Subjects may have difficulty acquiring the skill.
- It may be fatiguing for the weak or ill since sustained concentration is required to elicit the response.
- Patients with dyspnoea may not respond to a focus on breathing.
- Patients with cardiac irregularities may experience increased irregularity.
- Patients with low back pain may benefit more from strengthening their muscles rather than relaxing them.
- If used for more than two periods of 20–30 minutes daily some may experience withdrawal from life and symptoms ranging from insomnia to hallucinations.
- Psychotic patients may decompensate with profound relaxation
- Allergic or other adverse reactions may result if certain triggers are activated, e.g. picturing a corn field for a patient with hay fever.

Summary

The relaxation response is generally believed to have few if any negative effects, especially when relaxation is combined with visualization and providing both are competently taught and carried out. Perhaps the most cost-effective of all the complementary therapies, relaxation and visualization encourage patients to develop a sense of well-being and self-awareness. Self-healing results and the therapy can lead to personal development and growth.

REFERENCES

Benson H Klipper M Z 1977 The relaxation response. Collins, London

Chang J 1991 Using relaxation strategies in child and youth care practice. Child and Youth Care Forum 20: 155–169

Friedman S B Glasgow L A Ader R 1969 Psychosocial factors modifying host resistance to experimental infections. Annals of the New York Academy of Sciences 164: 381–393

Jacobson E 1977 You must relax, 5th edn. Souvenir Press, London

Meares A 1979 Strange places, simple truths. Collins, Glasgow

Patel C Marmot M G Terry D J et al 1985 Trial of relaxation in reducing coronary risk: four year follow up. British Medical Journal 290 (6475): 1103–1106

Reader's Digest Association 1991 Visualisation therapy; picturing your way to health. In: Reader's Digest family guide to alternative medicine. Reader's Digest Association, London

Ryman L 1994 Relaxation and visualisation. In: Wells R J Tschudin V (eds) Wells' supportive therapies in health care. Baillière Tindall, London

Selye H 1976 The stress of life, revised edn. McGraw-Hill, New York

Simonton O C Matthews-Simonton S Creighton J L 1978 Getting well again, a step-by-step, self-help guide to overcoming cancer for patients and their families. Bantam, London

Woodham A Peters D 1997 Encyclopaedia of complementary medicine. Dorling Kindersley, London

FURTHER READING – JOURNALS

Asaenok I S Spetsian L M Laysha N A 1988 Experience in using rooms for psycho-emotional relaxation at an engineering plant. Gigiena Truda i Professionalnye Zabolevaniia Jun 6: 50–51

Relaxation was found markedly to reduce the high fatigue levels felt at the end of the shift and also to bring about considerable reduction of the levels of irritation felt at work and disturbed sleep patterns.

Bullock E A Shaddy R E 1993 Relaxation and imagery techniques without sedation during right ventricular endomyocardial biopsy in pediatric heart transplant patients. Journal of Heart and Lung Transplantation 12: 59–62

Butler R J 1993 Establishing a dry run; a case study in securing bladder control. British Journal of Clinical Psychology 39: 215–217

Decker T W Cline-Elsen J 1992 Relaxation therapy as an adjunct in radiation oncology. Journal of Clinical Psychology 48: 388–393

Engel J M Rapoff M A Pressman A R 1992 Long-term follow-up of relaxation training for pediatric headache disorders. Headache 32: 152–156

Konno Y Ohno K 1987 A factor analytic study of the acceptance of relaxation through Dohsa training (psychological rehabilitation training). Shinrigaku Kenkyu (Japanese Journal of Psychology) 58: 57–61

This indicated amongst other things that willingness to apply oneself to the relaxation technique is indispensable for the required change.

Litchfield J 1993 Visualisation in coronary artery disease. Care of the Critically Ill 9: 35–36

Patel C Marmot M G Terry D J et al 1985 Trial of relaxation in reducing coronary risk: four year follow up. British Medical Journal 290 (6475): 1103–1106

Stephens R L 1992 Imagery: a treatment for nursing student anxiety. Journal of Nursing Education 31: 314–320

Zachariae R Kristensen J S Hokland P et al 1990 Effect of psychological intervention in the form of relaxation and guided imagery on cellular immune function in normal healthy subjects. An overview. Psychotherapy and Psychosomatics 54: 32–39

FURTHER READING – BOOKS

Chaitow L 1985 Your complete stress-proofing programme; how to protect yourself against the ill-effects of stress, including relaxation and meditation techniques. Thorsons, Wellingborough

Fleming U 1990 Grasping the nettle: a positive approach to pain. Collins Fount Paperbacks, London
Looks at the problem of pain in various forms (physical, mental and emotional) and shows a new way of learning how to live with it and overcome it.

Hewitt J 1992 The complete relaxation book. Rider.
Gawain S 1982 Creative visualisation. Bantam, New York
An introduction and work-book for the art of using mental energy to transform and greatly improve health, prosperity and loving relationships.

Madders J 1987 Stress and relaxation; self-help ways to cope with stress and relieve nervous tension, ulcers, insomnia, migraine and high blood pressure, 3rd edn. Macdonald Optima, London
Markham U 1989 The elements of visualisation. Element, Dorset
Describes visualization and looks at what it can do, what techniques are involved and how it can help improve our lives.

Tobias M Stewart M 1985 Stretch and Relax. Dorling Kindersley, London

USEFUL ADDRESSES

There is no governing body or national register of relaxation and visualization therapists. The Relaxation for Living Foundation (see below) provides courses for those wishing to learn to relax (using mainly physical exercise methods) and for those who wish to go on to teach others. A recent and exciting venture for nurses is an ENB course (see below) on stress management which has as one of its components relaxation.

British Holistic Medical Association
(BHMA)
179 Gloucester Place
London NW1 6DX
Tel: 020 7262 5299

English National Board for
Nursing, Midwifery and Health
Visiting (ENB)
170 Tottenham Court Road
London W1P 9LG
Stress management course for
nurses.

International Stress and Tension
Control Society (UK Branch)
The Priory Hospital
Priory Lane
Roehampton
London SW15 5JQ
Tel: 020 8876 8261

The Relaxation for Living Trust
Foxhills
30 Victoria Avenue
Shanklin
Isle of Wight
PO 37 6LS.
Information, courses, books
and tapes on relaxation for
stress management.

32 Shiatsu

Caroline Stevensen

Shiatsu – a hands-on therapy which works on energetic pathways to balance and heal the body.

'Shiatsu' means 'finger pressure' in Japanese but in practice it is much more than that. It is a therapy performed by the use of pressure from fingers, hands, elbows, knees and feet on the energetic pathways of the body called 'meridians'. It is along these meridians that the vital energy or life force of the body, known as 'Ki', flows. (Ki in Japanese is the same as Chi or Qi in Chinese.) Shiatsu aims to harmonize the Ki, promoting health and well-being throughout body, mind and spirit. It is traditionally performed on a padded mat or futon with the recipient clothed.

Shiatsu has its roots in oriental medicine and massage techniques dating back over 200 years. The modern form of shiatsu was introduced to the West only in the last 25 years (Gulliver et al 1993). It is a therapy which can be preventive as well as helpful in specific conditions. Through balancing the Ki, the recipient experiences relaxation and an improvement in many health problems. Shiatsu is a complementary therapy that can be given in conjunction with orthodox medical treatments as well as being a therapy in its own right. It combines diagnostic and treatment methods and encourages self-healing. It is being used increasingly in a wide variety of settings, but to date few nurses have undergone training.

HISTORICAL BACKGROUND

Massage, herbalism, acupuncture and moxibustion are all part of traditional Chinese medicine. The initial practice of massage in Japan known as 'Anma' resembles current Western massage in its active movements. Shiatsu, however, developed as a more subtle art involving the giving of still, relaxed pressure at defined points over the body (Lundberg 1992). It emerged from a manual therapy incorporating gentle manipulation, stretches and pressure techniques. It was recognized by the Japanese government as a therapy in its own right in the middle of the twentieth century (Lundberg 1992) and was brought to

Europe, USA, Australia and other parts of the Western world over the last 25 years where it is increasingly being used alongside orthodox health care.

Shiatsu is based on the 2000-year-old philosophy of traditional Chinese medicine (TCM). This states that from the universe or 'Tao', life energy made itself manifest in the forces of Yin and Yang, the positive and negative aspects of Ki. Ki flows through the body, supporting life and all its functions. The theory of Yin and Yang, the balance of opposite but complementary forces, was extended to include the Five Elements or Phases – Wood, Fire, Earth, Metal and Water – which influence the flow of Ki. On the basis of this complex system, definite characteristics were identified and associated with conditions of the body, illnesses or imbalances (Beresford-Cooke 1987). For example, the shouting quality in the voice and florid complexion of an alcoholic are related to disharmony in the Liver, ruled by the Wood element. TCM recognizes spiritual, mental, emotional and physical causes of disease and takes into account factors such as diet, exercise and other external influences, including climate. (See Chapter 15 on Acupuncture for further information on TCM theory.) Ki flows along the meridians defined in TCM and there have been some studies to support the existence of these energetic pathways (Becker 1976).

Styles of shiatsu

Various styles of shiatsu are practised in Japan and the West. These include zen shiatsu (most common), Tao shiatsu, seiki, macrobiotic shiatsu, healing shiatsu, Namikoshi shiatsu and hara shiatsu. The general principles previously mentioned apply to all approaches.

TREATMENT

Zen shiatsu involves the following sequence of events:

- History of the patient and his condition
- Diagnosis performed on the hara (abdomen) or back
- Delivery of the treatment
- Evaluation of the patient
- Recommendations to the patient.

History of the patient and his condition

An overall history of the patient is taken, including the well-being of body, mind and spirit. A medical history of the patient is taken which includes any illnesses and operations, medications, acute and chronic conditions and the patient's response to external factors such as food, weather, seasons of the year, times of the day and night, energy levels, general mood and, in the case of women, menstrual problems. The person's colouring, voice, posture and general attitude are also noted. Tongue and pulse diagnosis may be performed for a fuller understanding of the patient according to TCM.

Diagnosis performed on the hara or back

In shiatsu, visual diagnosis gives valuable information about the patient before any physical contact is made. Shiatsu diagnosis is performed on the hara (abdomen) or back by gentle palpation. The relative energetic qualities of the internal organs and their related meridians are assessed. Between the weakest, empty or most 'kyo' and the tightest, fullest or most 'jitsu' meridian, a reaction is felt by the practitioner which then guides the treatment.

Positioning of the patient

Shiatsu treatment is traditionally performed on a futon on the floor but can be given in a sitting position or on a treatment couch if the patient has difficulty getting down to floor level. A lower position makes it easier for the practitioner to provide pressure perpendicular to the meridian pathways with the help of gravity. The patient is fully clothed, preferably in a cotton tracksuit and socks. With the patient lying on his back, supported where necessary by pillows, the practitioner can observe the body for areas of tension and weakness. Any imbalance of Ki in the meridians as well as potential and existing health problems may be observed.

Delivery of the treatment

The principles in giving zen shiatsu are as follows (Masunaga & Ohashi 1977):

- Stationary perpendicular pressure: direct pressure is exerted at 90° to the meridian pathway.
- Penetration not pressure: pressure is exerted on the meridian point leaning with body weight and the help of gravity (not by physical force).
- Two-handed connectedness: both hands are used, one for support and the other to treat the meridian.
- Meridian continuity: the meridian is treated in its entirety to relieve any Ki blocked along its pathway and to give support as necessary.
- Relaxation of practitioner achieved by linking mind, hara and breath.

Intention and motivation are as important in shiatsu as any other therapy. The practitioner needs to remain relaxed and open to 'feel' what is happening to the patient. The focus of shiatsu is at the point on the hara called 'Tandien', the centre of balance and gravity, which is one centimetre below the umbilicus (Jarmey & Tschudin 1994). Shiatsu given from this point is relaxing and centring for the practitioner as well as the patient.

In shiatsu, treatment concentrates on the most kyo meridian, rather like supporting the weakest link in a chain. To begin, the 'supporting' hand is placed on the hara whilst the other hand 'palms' the leg along the weakest meridian pathway, feeling for imbalances in the Ki. The process is then repeated with the thumb, fingers, elbow or knee leaning in along the same meridian in order to balance the Ki. Along the meridians there are highly charged electromagnetic foci called 'tsubos' or pressure points (Ridolfi 1990) (these correspond to acupuncture points). The stimulation of the tsubos affects the meridian energy as well as energy in other parts of the body. By feeling the changing quality of the Ki along the meridian and in the tsubos the appropriate amount of pressure can be given to balance the energy. This process can then be repeated systematically around the body until the entire meridian system has been treated. The pressure of shiatsu should be deep but not overly painful. Blocked energy in a tsubo may feel painful and sensitive. Low energy may be felt deeper in the body. Recipients often describe a 'good hurt' in places where treatment is particularly needed. Pressures and stretches to other meridians are included in the treatment as appropriate. The whole body is worked on including the front, back, sides, limbs, neck and head, again according to individual need.

Evaluation of the patient

People commonly feel both invigorated and relaxed after shiatsu. An overall improvement in health and well-being is often felt before any change in a chronic condition. The eliminative channels of the body may need to be cleared before pain can be alleviated. Improvements on the physical, mental, emotional and spiritual levels are achieved with shiatsu. As with other such therapies, a 'healing reaction' may be provoked (Gulliver 1993). Long-standing stress, tension or a build-up of toxins may be released in the form of a slight aggravation of the condition or possibly 'flu like symptoms. This usually passes in less than 48 hours and an improvement is then felt.

Recommendations to the patient

Recommendations may include diet, exercise and lifestyle changes based on traditional Chinese medicine theory for the overall improvement of health, according to the individual.

Recent developments in shiatsu practice

Two students of Masunaga (1977) have taken the direction of shiatsu in different ways. In Tao shiatsu, Endo (1995) has developed the meridian system from Masunaga's 12 meridians to 24 throughout the body. He also works with other energy pathways that spiral through the body in different patterns. Indeed, the way that the meridian energy is contacted with touch and intention has a different emphasis than that used in other methods.

Another student of Masunaga, Kishi (personal communication) has developed a very subtle and spontaneous form of shiatsu, or it may be called a development from shiatsu called seiki. In seiki, the practitioner waits for the patient's energy to express its need to be worked with by the practitioner. In this form of treatment, the touch may be present or absent, using light or deep pressure, moving or stationary according to the needs of the patient.

Andrews (personal communication) who trained with Sasaki, a student of Masunaga, has also developed his own methods of vibrational shiatsu treatment, where the energetic needs of the client may be tuned into on spiritual, mental, emotional and physical levels. Also, the speed of vibration of the meridians may be tuned into in order to adjust the speed of treatment to be in harmony with the patient. Inner sound may also be used by the practitioner to enhance the rebalancing and retuning of the meridians, as with a musical instrument.

These advanced shiatsu methods offer further degrees of fine tuning for the practitioner, allowing treatments to be more directed to the needs of the patient. In this way there is a greater effectiveness possible for the treatment as the attention of the practitioner may be focused and tuned in ways to best meet the needs of the patient. In all shiatsu training, self-development is extremely important as the sensitivity and awareness of the practitioner is key to the effectiveness of the treatment.

Therapeutic potential in nursing

The main aims of shiatsu are as follows (Jarmey & Tschudin 1994):
- To promote relaxation
- To improve blood and lymphatic flow
- To alleviate aches and pains
- To provide empathy and support
- To heighten bodily awareness.

The conditions most amenable to treatment by shiatsu and of therapeutic benefit in nursing are (Ridolfi 1990):
- headaches and migraine

Therapeutic potential in nursing (Cont'd)

- respiratory illnesses including asthma and bronchitis
- sinus trouble with catarrh
- insomnia and restlessness
- circulatory problems
- anxiety and tension
- depression and other psychological problems
- fatigue and lethargy
- somatic disturbances resulting from mental problems
- digestive disorders
- bowel problems
- low libido
- painful menstruation
- pregnancy and childbirth
- urogenital conditions
- rheumatic and arthritic complaints
- back trouble, including sciatica
- following sprains and strains and other injuries, but not in first 24 hours due to pain and swelling
- integration of physical, mental, emotional and spiritual aspects.

To say that shiatsu can be helpful for any condition may be a little broad but certainly in improving overall well-being, promoting calm, rest and relaxation, it can enhance quality of life for most people. Indeed, shiatsu can be ideal for maintaining good health. Although conditions are treated according to oriental diagnosis with shiatsu, western medical diagnosis can be taken into account.

Contraindications for use

As shiatsu works directly on the body, the contraindications for general massage apply. Do not treat:

- Osteoporosis, fractures and bony metastases due to pressure
- Burns, wounds, broken skin, infectious skin diseases
- Unexplained swellings
- Operation sites for at least 1–2 months
- Directly over varicose veins
- Low platelet count, tendency to easy bruising, over present bruising
- High fevers, as touch is generally not tolerated
- Contagious diseases due to infection risk
- Lower legs and specifically contraindicated points in the first trimester of pregnancy, especially if there is a history of spontaneous abortion

Contraindications for use (Cont'd)

- With immune deficiency problems including AIDS, ME and cancer, lighter techniques and shorter treatments may be used so as not to exhaust the patient
- Cardiac or chronic respiratory patients in the prone position, unless an exact knowledge of their current status is known
- On the head with epileptics or with blood pressure > 200 mmHg systolic.

Summary

Shiatsu is a deep and effective hands-on treatment for many conditions as well as being very relaxing and providing support for general health and well-being. Through the balancing of the body's energy, better physiological and psychological functioning can occur. Recommendations for diet and lifestyle based on TCM theory can also be offered, according to individual need. The 3-year part-time training in shiatsu is demanding but enables the nurse using shiatsu to offer a particularly beneficial complementary therapy.

REFERENCES

Becker R, Marino A, Spadaro J 1976 Electrophysiological correlates of acupuncture points and meridians. Psychoenergetic Systems 1: 105–112
Beresford-Cooke C 1987 Shiatsu. In: Lidell L (ed) The book of massage. Ebury Press, London
Endo R 1995 Tao shiatsu. Japan Publications Inc., Tokyo
Gulliver N, Liechti E, Lunberg P 1993 A guide to shiatsu. Shiatsu Society, Wokingham
Jarmey C, Tschudin V 1994 Shiatsu. In: Wells R, Tschudin V (eds) Wells' supportive therapies in health care. Baillière Tindall, London
Lundberg P 1992 The book of shiatsu. Gaia Books, London
Masunaga S, Ohashi W 1977 Zen shiatsu. Japan Publications, New York
Ridolfi R 1990 Alternative health: shiatsu. Optima, London

FURTHER READING – JOURNALS

Formby J 1997 Shiatsu massage for carers. Complementary Therapies in Medicine 5 (1): 47–48
Harris P, Pooley N 1998 What do shiatsu practitioners treat? A nationwide survey. Complementary Therapies in Medicine 6 (1): 45–46
Stevensen C 1995 The role of shiatsu in palliative care. Complementary Therapies in Nursing and Midwifery 1: 51–58

FURTHER READING – BOOKS

Beresford-Cooke C 1996 Shiatsu theory and practice. Churchill Livingstone, Edinburgh

Jarmey C, Tindall J 1991 Acupressure for common ailments. Gaia Books, London

Kaptchuk T J 1989 Chinese medicine: the web that has no weaver. Rider, London

Maciocia G 1989 The foundations of Chinese medicine. Churchill Livingstone, London

Ohashi W 1988 Do-it-yourself shiatsu. Unwin Paperbacks, London

USEFUL ADDRESSES

Shiatsu Society
Barber House
Storeys Bar Road
Fengate
Peterborough
PE1 5YS

Tel 01733 758 341
Fax 01733 758 342
E-mail: admin@shiatsu.org
Website: www.shiatsu.org

Therapeutic touch

Jean Sayre-Adams

Therapeutic touch – *an energy field interaction between two or more people, aimed at rebalancing or repatterning the energy field to promote relaxation and pain relief and activate self-healing.*

The use of touch in the act of laying on of hands is one of the oldest therapies known to humans. Therapeutic touch (TT) is a modern form of the laying on of hands, and the name originates from Dr Dolores Kreiger, Professor of Nursing at New York University. The concepts that form its foundations are both simple and complex and can be found at the cutting edge of modern physics (Capra 1976, Booth 1993).

The theoretical concepts of TT have previously been linked to the eastern ideas of chakras and meridians (Govinda 1974, Krieger 1993). More recently the theoretical basis of TT has become closely associated with Martha Rogers' nursing theory – the Science of Unitary Human Beings (Rogers 1970) and consequently with relativity theory and quantum theory (Lutjens 1991). Rogers' Science of Unitary Human Beings appears to have originated approximately 30 years ago in her early writings (Lutjens 1991). She perceived nursing as a unique science, conceptually distinct from any other science. The Science of Unitary Human Beings is described as a synthesis of facts and ideas to create a unique way of perceiving people and their environment. The fulcrum of the theory is the uniqueness of human beings and their interactions with the world. This focus upon individuals is presented as underpinning the practice of nursing.

Lutjens (1991) describes Rogers' central theme as that of acausality in an infinite universe of open systems; i.e. there is no such thing as cause-and-effect since this implies a beginning and an end. In contrast to a linear approach to health care, Rogers views existence and our interactions with all things as being in a continual state of change. Drawing on Heisenberg's principle of uncertainty and on quantum theory she describes our world as an energy system. This energy is never stable but in continual flow and ebb – creating and recreating patterns, oscillating between balance and imbalance, health and illness. Human beings are seen as dynamic energy fields. Rogers' theory is continually evolving and developing but the basis of this approach is briefly as follows:

- Energy – energy fields are the fundamental units of all living things (Rogers 1990).

- Human beings are whole entities and should never be perceived simply in terms of their parts.

- Humans as energy fields are continually and simultaneously exchanging energy with one another and with the environment.

- Each energy field has a unique pattern, rather like a finger print.

- Individual energy fields are in a continual process of interaction with the environment. Thus, even a repeated action is not the same; time has moved on and our energy has imperceptibly altered. One never walks the same stream twice (Lutjens 1990).

- Although unique, each energy field is constantly changing, like a wave in the sea.

- The energy field extends to many other dimensions in addition to the three-dimensional world; this is referred to as 'pandimensionality'.

In recent years there have been suggestions that the Science of Unitary Human Beings is congruent with TT and Rogers' approach is increasingly referred to when explaining therapeutic touch. Therapeutic touch works on the premiss that all individuals are unique energy fields. Imbalances or disruptions in the flow of energy can be rebalanced or repatterned by the therapist towards a state of harmony and balance. TT is a specific therapeutic modality and is distinct from any other forms of energy healing (Quinn 1993).

Although there has been much research on TT (Quinn 1988), it is still not clearly understood how TT works. Quinn (1992) suggests a repatterning of the energy field of the person in imbalance is being initiated by the therapist, and influenced by the therapist's centred state and energy field.

HISTORICAL BACKGROUND

Although TT is a relatively new modality, healing through touch is probably as old as civilization itself. Evidence of the use of touch to promote well-being can be found in cave drawings. The oldest written documentation of healing with touch comes from the Orient 5000 years ago. It has been used in all cultures: Egyptian, Chinese, Indian, Polynesian, native American Indian, Greek and Roman (Turton 1988, Booth 1993, Harvey 1983). The Bible tells of healing through touch performed by Christ (Turton 1988). Touch was widely used by shamans and traditional practitioners until the rise of the Puritan culture during the 1600s. With the development of Christianity, Turton (1988) notes that healing was claimed as the domain of the clergy and this restricted widespread use. Touch as a healing art remained relatively unacknowledged until research into its benefits began in the 1950s (Dossey et al 1988, Sayre-Adams & Wright 1995).

In the late 1960s, Dr Dolores Krieger, Professor of Nursing at New York University, learned the laying on of hands from Dora Kunz (Kunz 1991) and over the next several years practised and promoted therapeutic touch within nursing. In the early 1970s, Krieger began to teach TT to her Master's degree students in a class entitled 'Frontiers in nursing'. TT is now mainstream nursing practice in the USA.

TREATMENT

The aim of a TT treatment is to rebalance or repattern the energy field of the patient, therefore bringing relaxation and facilitating the healing process. TT can be carried out in any setting that the practitioner feels is appropriate, for example, a quiet room in a hospital, in a garden, or at home. First, the practitioner centres him- or herself, in order to become harmonious with the patient. At this time the intention to help is also reaffirmed. An assessment of the patient is then made by the practitioner by moving her hands over the entire energy field. The practitioner returns to the areas where an imbalance has been felt and, continuing to use the hands, rebalances or repatterns the field.

Stages of technique

Centring – the practitioner becomes relaxed, calm and focused on the care about to be given.

Assessment – the practitioner places her hands close to the client's body and gently moves them over the body. The aim is to identify subtle changes in the body's energy.

Treatment – the practitioner focuses attention on specific areas of the body in order to rebalance and redirect energy.

Evaluation – the point at which the practitioner considers sufficient treatment has been given.

Therapeutic potential in nursing

Research on therapeutic touch has shown it to be effective for:

- pain relief
- anxiety
- loneliness (in the elderly)

Therapeutic potential in nursing (cont'd)

- rehabilitation
- wound healing
- headaches
- insomnia
- hypertension
- increased haemoglobin count
- relaxation
- stress-related anxiety (see contraindications).

Clinical practice suggests it may complement care in the following:

- upper respiratory infections
- allergies
- musculoskeletal conditions
- well-being of neonates (see contraindications)
- labour and delivery (see contraindications)
- nausea
- fatigue
- comfort of the dying
- lowering temperatures
- premenstrual syndrome
- secondary, opportunistic infections of AIDS
- shingles
- the promotion of emotional and spiritual well-being.

Contraindications for use

Situations in which one must proceed with extra sensitivity and limit treatment to shorter periods are as follows:

- babies
- frail elderly
- pregnant women
- head injuries
- emaciated patients
- psychosis
- shock.

Intentionality and centredness are the two most important qualities in a practitioner. If the practitioner is not able to become and stay centred or if they do not have the intention to help, then TT will be ineffective and the practitioner may feel drained and unwell.

Summary

Therapeutic touch is a common part of nursing practice in North America (Sayre-Adams 1993) and interest in and commitment to it has grown among nurses in the UK. TT has the potential to become integrated within mainstream nursing practice since it offers another dimension in healing and caring. Research so far suggests that TT can bring significant benefits to patients, at minimal cost. However, greater understanding of Rogers' theory as well as continued and replicated studies on TT by nurses are needed (Quinn 1989).

REFERENCES

Booth B 1993 Complementary therapy. Macmillan, London

Capra F 1976 Tao of physics. Bantam, New York

Dossey B Keegan L Guzzetta C Gooding Kolkmeier L 1988 Holistic nursing: a handbook for practice. Aspen, Gaitherburg, MD

Govinda L A 1974 Foundations of Tibetan mysticism. Weiser, New York

Harvey D 1983 The power to heal: an investigation of healing and the healing experience. The Aquarian Press, London

Krieger D 1993 Accepting your power to heal. Bear, Santa Fe, NM

Kunz D 1991 The personal aura. Quest, Wheaten, IL

Lutjens L R J 1991 Martha Rogers. The Science of Unitary Human Beings. Notes on nursing theories. Sage, Newbury Park, CA

Quinn J F 1988 Building a body of knowledge. Journal of Holistic Nursing 6: 37–45

Quinn J F 1989 Future directions for Therapeutic Touch research. Journal of Holistic Nursing 7: 19–25

Quinn J F 1992 Holding sacred space: the nurse as healing environment. Holistic Nursing Practice 6: 26–36

Quinn J F 1993 Psychoimmunologic effects of Therapeutic Touch on practitioners and recently bereaved recipients: a pilot study. Advances in Nursing Science 15: 13–26

Rogers M 1970 An introduction to the theoretical basis of nursing. FA Davis, Philadelphia

Sayre-Adams J 1993 Therapeutic Touch – principles and practice. Complementary Therapies in Medicine 1: 96–99

Sayre-Adams J Wright S 1995 Theory and practice of Therapeutic Touch. Churchill Livingstone, Edinburgh

Turton P 1988 Healing: Therapeutic Touch. In: Rankin-Box D F (ed) Complementary health therapies: a guide for nurses and the caring professions. Croom Helm, Beckenham, Kent

FURTHER READING – JOURNALS

There is a large body of research on TT, much of it conducted in the US. An extended compendium of TT research can be requested from The Sacred Space Foundation

Biley F 1992 The science of unitary human beings: a contemporary literature review. Nursing Practice 15: 23–26

Heidt P R 1991 Helping patients to rest: clinical studies in Therapeutic Touch. Holistic Nursing Practice 5: 57–66

Kramer N A 1990 Comparison of Therapeutic Touch and casual touch in stress reduction of hospitalised children. Paediatric Nursing 16: 483–485

Meehan T C 1993 Therapeutic Touch and post-operative pain: a Rogerian research study. Nursing Science Quarterly 6: 69–77

Quinn J F 1984 Therapeutic Touch as energy exchange: testing the theory. Advances in Nursing Science 6: 42–49

Quinn J F 1989 Therapeutic Touch as energy exchange: replication and extension. Nursing Science Quarterly 2: 79–87

Sayre-Adams J 1994 Therapeutic Touch: a nursing function. Nursing Standard 8: 25–28

Winstead-Fry P, Kÿek J 1999 An interogative review and meta-analysis of therapeutic touch research. Alternative Therapies in Health and Medicine 5(6): 58–67

Wirth D P Richardson J T Eidelman W S O'Malley A C 1993 Full thickness dermal wounds treated with non-contact Therapeutic Touch: a replication and extension. Complementary Therapies in Medicine 1: 127–132

FURTHER READING – BOOKS

Krieger D 1979 The Therapeutic Touch: how to use your hands to help or heal. Prentice Hall, Englewood Cliffs, NJ

Macrae J 1988 Therapeutic Touch: a practical guide. Arcana, London

Meehan T C 1990 The science of unitary human beings and theory-based practice: Therapeutic Touch. In: Barrett E A M (ed) Visions of Rogers' science based nursing. National League for Nursing, New York

Rogers M E 1990 Nursing: Science of unitary irreducible human beings: update 1990. In: Barrett E A M (ed) Visions of Rogers' science based nursing. National League for Nursing, New York, p 5–11

Talbot M 1991 The holographic universe. Harper Collins, New York

Wright S, Sayre - Adams J 2000 Sacred space: right relationship and spirituality in health care. Churchill Livingstone, Edinburgh

USEFUL ADDRESSES

ENB accredited courses are available from the Sacred Space Foundation. The regulatory body for TT in the UK is the British Association of Therapeutic Touch.

British Association of Therapeutic Touch
Redmire
Mungrisdale
Cumbria CA11 0TB

International Society of Rogerian Scholars

School of Nursing Studies (Mr Fran Biley)
University of Wales College of Medicine
Heath Park
Cardiff CF4 4XN
Tel: 029 2081 0895

Sacred Space Foundation
Highland Hall
Renwick
Penrith
Cumbria CA10 1JL
Tel: 01768 898375

Glossary

Acupuncture – derived from the Latin words *acus* (needle) and *punctara* (puncture). Chinese medical system which aims to diagnose illness and promote health by stimulating the body's self-healing powers.

Alexander technique – psychophysical postural re-education. Posture is perceived as an important contributor to health. The technique seeks to provide a process of postural re-education in order to encourage individuals to monitor consciously how they use their bodies. Thus, the technique suggests that bodily posture has an effect on physical and psychological well-being. By re-educating individuals in both posture and use of their bodies, physical and psychological well-being can be enhanced.

Aromatherapy – a form of treatment using essential oils extracted from plants which may be inhaled or massaged into the skin for therapeutic effects.

Autogenic training – a psychophysiological form of psychotherapy, conducted by the client which involves passive concentration upon particular combinations of psychophysiological verbal stimuli. It is designed as a self-care tool.

Bach flower remedies – the use of the distilled essences of wild flowers taken diluted in water or as a lotion. The therapy is based on the premiss that disease is directly related to temperament; thus remedies treat, for example, anxiety, insomnia, disharmony.

Biofeedback – a method of training designed to enable an individual to control involuntary bodily functions, usually with the assistance of electronic equipment.

Centring – an initial stage of preparation by the practitioner in which she becomes relaxed, calm and focused on the care about to be given. This activity is described by a number of therapies, e.g. therapeutic touch and shiatsu.

Chiropractic – specializes in the diagnosis and treatment of mechanical disorders of joints and their effects on the nervous system. The spine is afforded particular attention. Displacement of spinal vertebrae may result in the manifestion of a range of seemingly unrelated symptoms. The aim of chiropractic is not to treat the symptoms but to identify the subluxation and correct it manually.

Clearing – a gentle sweeping action whereby the practitioner moves her hands over the client's body in an attempt to smooth or rebalance the energy field (see Therapeutic Touch).

Colour therapy – the use of colour in lighting, paints or materials to correct physical and psychological problems.

Counselling skills – a repertoire of learnt behaviours, both verbal and non-verbal. Adopting these skills enables a rapport to be established, facilitating the communication process.

Crystal therapy – grounded in the belief that minerals and rocks possess therapeutic forms of energy; for example, crystal creates harmony, malachite resolves inflammation.

EDR – electrodermal response, registers general levels of autonomic arousal (see Biofeedback).

Essential oil – Undiluted oil extracted from plants and commonly diluted in a carrier oil before use.

GSR – galvanic skin response, registers levels of autonomic arousal (see Biofeedback).

Geopathic stress – Based on the concept that energies emanate from the earth, which may affect general health and well-being.

Hara diagnosis – a form of diagnosis used in shiatsu involving gentle palpation of the abdominal region. The focus of shiatsu is at the point on the hara known as tandien, the centre of balance and gravity.

Healing – a therapeutic form of energy exchange that may occur between two or more individuals with the conscious intention to improve health and well-being.

Herbal medicine – the use of whole plant material by trained practitioners to promote recovery from disease and to enable healing to take place.

Homeopathy – a system of medicine based upon the Law of Similars (let like be treated with like). Effectivity is obtained by the process of dilution, in which extracts from natural sources such as plants and minerals are diluted many times in a water and alcohol base. At each dilution the mixture is vigorously shaken, a process known as succussion. It is this process which homeopaths believe initiates the healing potency of the dilution.

Humour and laughter therapy – a humorous or amusing intervention used by the health care professional or patient and designed to be of benefit to the patient.

Hypnosis – in health care, the deliberate use of the trance state to enhance the sense of health and well-being.

Iridology – a diagnostic tool based on the assumption that the iris can indicate the general status of internal organs. Iridology may be used by herbalists and naturopaths.

Kinesiology – a therapy that tests different muscles to identify and/or prevent allergies.

Massage – the conscious, deliberate and often formalized use of the instinctive response to comfort another person by touch.

Meridians – conceptual channels along which Qi energy flows in the body (see Acupuncture and Shiatsu).

Music therapy – The use of music in order to enhance, improve and maintain physical, emotional and spiritual well-being.

Nutritional therapy – based on the assumption that the state of one's health is directly contingent upon what is eaten. Nutritional therapy focuses upon the effects certain foods have on health and well-being.

Naturopathy – a multidisciplinary approach to health care founded on a belief in the power of the body to heal itself.

Osteopathy – A system of manual medicine concerned with mechanical, functional and postural assessment and treatment. This usually involves manipulation of joints and spinal vertebrae directed towards resolving mechanical problems of the body. Thus abnormal tension in muscles and ligaments can be relieved and self-healing facilitated.

Placebo response – a self-healing response.

Process of counselling – occurs within a non-directive therapeutic relationship, whereby the client will be enabled to self-actualize and develop his own abilities to resolve or accept his situation.

Radionics – based on the concept that each part of the body vibrates at specific rates. In illness the vibrations alter. Changes can be corrected with instruments that send back energy to the affected organs. Treatment can be done using blood or hair samples without the presence of the client.

Reflexology – a treatment which applies varying degrees of pressure to different parts of the body, commonly the hands and feet, in order to promote health and well-being. It is suggested that there are reflexes or zones running along the body and terminating in the hands or feet. All systems and organs are said to be reflected on to the hands or feet and by applying gentle pressure to specific areas of the hands or feet a change can be effected elsewhere in the body.

Relaxation – a state of consciousness characterized by feelings of peace and release from tension, anxiety and fear.

Shiatsu – literally means 'finger pressure'. A hands-on therapy which works on the energetic pathways to balance and strengthen the body in order to facilitate self-healing.

Succussion – used in homeopathy, a process whereby natural diluted substances are vigorously shaken. Homeopaths believe that it is this process that facilitates the healing potential of the dilution.

Target organ – term used in biofeedback to describe the organ or part of the body from which changing levels of activity can be demonstrated, for example skin, brain, heart.

Therapeutic touch (TT) – described as an energy field interaction between two or more people with the intention to rebalance or repattern the energy field in order to facilitate relaxation and self-healing.

Trance – an altered state of consciousness.

Visualization – the technique of using the imagination to create any desired changes in an individual's life.

Yin/Yang – represents the dynamic balance of energy. Yang energy is characterized by heat, movement, activity and excess; Yin energy relates more to cold, sluggishness, inactivity and deficiency. A balance of each kind of energy is necessary for health.

Zones – a term used in reflexology. It is suggested that the body's innate energy flows through reflexes or zones which terminate in the hands or feet.

Additional addresses

Alexander technique

Society of Teachers of the
Alexander Technique (STAT)
20 London House
266 Fulham Road
London SW10 9EL
Tel: 020 7351 0828

Chiropractic

British Chiropractic Association
29 Whitley Street
Reading
Berkshire RG2 0EG
Tel: 0118 950 5950

Scottish Chiropractic Association
16 Jenny Moores Road
St Boswells
Roxburghshire
Scotland TO6 0AL
Tel: 01835 824026

Osteopathy

General Osteopathic Council
Osteopathy House
176 Tower Bridge Road
London SE1 3LU
Tel: 020 7357 6655

Cranial Osteopathic Association
478 Baker Street
Enfield
Middlesex EN1 3QS
Tel: 020 8367 5561

Natural Therapeutic and
Osteopathic Society and Register
168 High Street
Maldon
Essex CM2 7BX
Tel: 01621 859094

Feng Shui

Feng Shui Network International
8 Kings Court
Pateley Bridge
Harrogate
North Yorkshire
HG3 5JW

Research and education sources

Association of Medical Research
Charities (AMRC)
29–35 Farringdon Road
London ECM 3JB
UK
Tel: 020 7404 6454
Fax: 020 7404 6448
E-mail: amrc@mailbox.ulcc.ac.uk.
Website: http://www.amrc.org.uk

Foundation for Integrated Medicine
International House
50 Compton Road
London N1 2YT
UK
Tel: 020 7688 1881
Fax: 020 7688 1882
E-mail: enquiries@fimed.org
Website: www.fimed.org

Complementary Therapies in
Nursing Forum
Royal College of Nursing (RCN)
20 Cavendish Square
London W1M 0AB
Tel: 020 7409 3333

Complementary Therapies in
Nursing and Midwifery
PO Box 10
Macclesfield
Cheshire SK10 4HW

E-mail:
drankinbox@compuserve.com
Tel: 01625 820898
Fax: 01625 820029
Website: http://www.harcourt-
international.com/journals/ctnm

Medical Research Council
20 Park Crescent
London W1N 4AL
Tel: 020 7636 5422

Institute for Complementary
Medicine
PO Box 194
London SE16 7QZ
Tel: 020 7237 5165
Fax: 020 7237 5175
ICM –
website: www.icmedicine.co.uk

Centre for the Study of
Complementary Medicine
51 Bedford Place
Southampton
Hampshire SO1 2DG
Tel: 023 8033 4752

Council for Complementary and
Alternative Medicine
Suite D
Park House
206–208 Latimer Road
London W10 6RC.

Confederation of Healing
Organizations
Suite J, 2nd Floor
The Red and White House
113 High Street
Berkhampstead
Hertfordshire HP4 2DJ
Tel: 01442 870660

Sacred Space Foundation
Redmire
Mungrisdale
Cumbria CA11 0TB
Tel: 01768 779000
Fax: 01768 779111

Index

Page numbers in *italics* refer to boxes, *g* indicates a glossary definition.